From North Korea
to America
Through Three Wars

From North Korea to America Through Three Wars
A Nurse's Journey

Sung C. Yoo

Foreword by Lynn Hamilton
Introduction by E. Taylor Atkins
Afterword by Heeyoung Choi

McFarland & Company, Inc., Publishers
Jefferson, North Carolina

ISBN (print) 978-1-4766-9792-5
ISBN (ebook) 978-1-4766-5585-7

Library of Congress cataloging data are available

Library of Congress Control Number 2025019758

© 2025 Sung C. Yoo. All rights reserved

No part of this book may be reproduced or transmitted in any form or by any means, electronic or mechanical, including photocopying or recording, or by any information storage and retrieval system, without permission in writing from the publisher.

Front cover images: Sung C. Yoo as nursing manager at Merwick Care & Rehabilitation Center (early 2003). *Background* "Land in Peace" by Len Yoo.

Printed in the United States of America

McFarland & Company, Inc., Publishers
Box 611, Jefferson, North Carolina 28640
www.mcfarlandpub.com

To my brother, Sung Kul, who made me a nurse;
my supportive husband, Insok;
and all my lovely children, 현주 (Julie), 효민 (Peggy), and 한스 (Hans);
and to Kenton Clymer for his tireless assistance in building this book
and making a long dream of mine possible. Without him,
this book would not have taken shape.

Table of Contents

Acknowledgments	ix
Foreword: Sung C. Yoo and the Evolution of a Professional Identity BY LYNN HAMILTON	1
Introduction: Sung C. Yoo's Place in History BY E. TAYLOR ATKINS	13
Prologue: An Unexpected Moment	29
I—Leaving North Korea	31
II—The Forgotten War in South Korea	42
III—The Reluctant Nursing Student	59
IV—The Vietnam War	67
V—Seeking the American Dream	96
VI—Florence Nightingale	116
VII—Mother, Grandmother, Sister, Counselor, Teacher, Nurse	127
VIII—Final Reflections	141
Afterword: Navigating the Historical and Sociopolitical Intersection of Nurse Migration BY HEEYOUNG CHOI	149
Chapter Notes	163
Index	171

Acknowledgments

This book was born after a conversation in Palm Springs in 2020. I am most grateful for the support, encouragement, advice, and help from many people. The debt owed to those who gave not just sufficiently but lavishly is crystal clear. Usic Kim, professor of sociology at Ewha Womans University, planted the seed to develop my writing skills and continually helped me to improve. He read drafts of my story many times, made spelling corrections, added the names of persons and places, and identified correct years and locations. He urged me to write a memoir, and he is the person most delighted to see this memoir in print.

Lynn Hamilton, a former nurse in the U.S. Army during the Vietnam War, now retired from the University of Michigan as an educational nurse specialist, is the foundational base of this book. After she read the first of my poor paragraphs, she made the difference between the sky and the earth. And then she strongly encouraged me with no hesitations because she was impressed by my efforts and survival. Her compassion overflowed from her heart. Kenton Clymer, distinguished research professor of history emeritus at Northern Illinois University, was the coordinator for this book. He has been my teacher, supporter, guide, energy supplier, builder, and adviser for the whole book. I have learned from him more than I can express in a single word. Never before in my 86 years have I had help extended with a pure heart and mind and intelligence. I dream of being like him.

Heeyoung Choi, a recent PhD graduate from Northern Illinois University, read the entire story and urged me to continue writing. The encouragement and support from this young Korean woman was unbelievable. She was humble and pure and a scholar

Acknowledgments

in cultural history and women's studies. Her help was deeply appreciated, as is the afterword she contributed to this book. Elizabeth Keech, professor of nursing at Villanova University, now retired and an adjunct professor of nursing, read the entire story, revised spelling and grammatical mistakes, helped with appropriate vocabulary and idioms, and always encouraged and supported my efforts to continue. E. Taylor Atkins, distinguished teaching professor of history at Northern Illinois University, selflessly took the time to write the introduction, which placed everything in its historical context. Thanks, Taylor.

Mary Boylston, retired professor of nursing at Eastern University, recognized my unique story and recommended an English-language editor to complete the work. Ronald Stone, professor emeritus of Christian ethics at Pittsburgh Theological Seminary and recently the author of distinguished books about theologians Reinhold Niebuhr and Paul Tillich, read the entire story with sincerity and commented and edited it, always offering concrete support and encouragement. He suggested more focus on nursing. Tisha S. Woo, user services librarian at the Clifford E. Barbour Library, Pittsburgh Theological Seminary, kindly helped and assisted me in finding references and maps as well as sending pictures and providing help with other computer skills.

My friend Evalynn Welling read the entire book with much curiosity because of her feelings about the wars and particularly because of her connections with the war in Ukraine. This in turn increased my own desire to write. Sean Skulski was an exceptional editor with great humor and cheerful comments who notably improved the final product. Simon Hebert was my essential computer teacher. He helped me navigate old and newer computers with patience and in general helped my writing skills. He provided emotional support that enabled me to proceed with the writing. His calmness and excellent computer skills were of great value.

A special appreciation to W.D. Ehrhart, one of the best soldier writers to emerge from the war in Vietnam, for his assistance in contacting McFarland and to Sophia Lyons at McFarland, who has guided us through the publication process with skill and grace.

Finally, my greatest gratitude goes to my family: to my brother,

Acknowledgments

Sung Kul, who persisted in urging me to become a nurse; to my loving husband, Insok Yoo, who always supported me in writing this memoir in spite of the many hours that it took; and to all of my children, who are very proud that I was able to write this story for them and my grandchildren, while also learning something about Korean history. Their love and support gave me great comfort.

Foreword

Sung C. Yoo and the Evolution of a Professional Identity

by Lynn Hamilton

How improbable, on a golden afternoon in Palm Springs, California, to linger over a long lunch hearing firsthand about a lifetime of extraordinary struggle. Sung C. Yoo and I met in January 2020 just before the Covid epidemic sheltered us and the world. We were "snowbirds," it turned out, spending a season away from chillier climes. Our mutual friend, Molly Mowat, had a special interest in Sung's origin because Molly's own husband, Don, had more than once put himself at risk in devotion to help people inside North Korea. Knowing Sung and I each had experiences related to nursing care in the Vietnam era, Molly hosted us that day.

I had never knowingly encountered anyone born in North Korea, nor had I ever really talked with anyone having lived through childhood and grown up in the midst of war. Once we started, we engaged over an entire afternoon. How amazing: a vibrant and glowing yet delicate 80-plus-year-old describing some of the worst personal struggles and background. As her story unfolded, my sister—nurse Marlee Clymer—and I found ourselves probing for more. At every turn, we knew we were hearing an extraordinary story from an equally extraordinary woman. We knew it was a story worth writing. Our luncheon stretched to dinnertime.

Sung Yoo's is an exceptional memoir of continual personal stumbling blocks, a life that ultimately results in personal and professional

Foreword

transformation, achievement, and—ultimately—a complete professional paradigm shift. In vivid emotional detail, she brings us along as she describes many of her uphill emotional battles—how she overcomes, moves to the next barrier, wrestles with it, and finds her own self-willed path through it. The story itself is incredible: a harrowing childhood escape from North Korea; the miseries of life in 1950s South Korea as war came there; the longing for dignity and self-sustenance for the future, yet resistance to a brotherly prescribed solution; the necessity to earn sufficient money that drove a young couple to sacrifice in order to earn enough in Vietnam during war there; the difficulties encountered after a move to America for a better life; the hard-won ultimate resolution. It's a profoundly moving, sometimes breathtaking, and often poignant story.

An element that makes the story especially revealing is the degree of self-reflection interspersed at every stage. Sung challenges herself, opens herself emotionally, never holds back. From a human perspective, this is remarkable. Sung's narrative is guileless, open, honest, and relatable as she endures experiences that those of us who are otherwise comfortable in the world would find *unrelatable*.

In telling her story, Sung Yoo raises multiple issues of concern even today: class, race, cultural barriers and sensitivities; nursing as a way out of poverty; the changing attitudes toward nursing as a profession; self-identity and personal and professional transformation. All of these thread throughout the narrative, with different insights at different stages of her life. All reflect a pattern of growth and self-actualization.

Sung Yoo and I Share a Vietnam War History

Sung and I are both nurses, baccalaureate prepared, who have treated Vietnam War casualties—yet the circumstances were completely different! Desperation drove Sung to choose nursing in the first place. Having experienced the ravages of two wars while growing up, she was driven by continual financial pressures to another war zone again as a young adult early in a nursing career and ultimately to emigrate to the United States in 1970.

Sung C. Yoo and the Evolution of a Professional Identity

As a new college graduate with a bachelor's in nursing, in 1966, I was without any financial encumberment thanks to an upper-middle-class suburban upbringing. Always intending to venture from home for the wider world, I chose to leave an initial, well-paid local hospital staff nurse job for a belief in "contributing to the war effort" and the novelty of travel and living in a new country. In a two-year "guaranteed assignment program" available through the U.S. Army Nurse Corps at the time, I knew that, living in Japan, I would never be in physical danger as in Vietnam; Sung Yoo chose her assignment in Vietnam despite the probable physical danger and, as it turned out, was definitely in great jeopardy. We both felt the pressure and stresses of experiencing dreadful casualties, but mine were within a safe personal context. Hers were close to the action, putting her in personal danger. There was no comparison.

Thousands of miles apart and unbeknownst to each other, Sung and I were treating our different, respective patient populations. Mine were all U.S. soldiers in a 1,000-bed U.S. Army hospital (the 106th General, Yokohama) devoted entirely to Vietnam casualties. After rescue and initial care in Vietnam followed by air force medical evacuation of four to six hours, seriously injured patients were ferried the last leg to our hospital. Our mission was to treat and stabilize patients—ideally to send them back to war, but if not (and mostly not), then to get them well enough to withstand the trip back to the States. My own work area, the Burn Unit, extended the entire length of a second floor—four big, open "wards," some 60 beds total. Burns of all kinds—explosions, accidents, napalm; first to third degree; small or full body—all were funneled to one particular place, my unit. Burn injuries demand specialized care. In time, ours became an extension of the Brooke Army Burn Center at Fort Sam Houston, San Antonio.

The Tet Offensive of January 1968 began Sung's year in Vietnam and my second year in Japan. What a dramatic change for us both. For me, suddenly the pace picked up. Increasingly, the sound of helicopters on the adjacent landing pad became a continual thwacking, the noise portending another dreadful influx of seriously injured soldiers. By necessity, I joined other team members working 12-hour shifts, six days a week, for the rest of my time that year. Meanwhile, in Vietnam, in the thick of the increased war activity, Sung Yoo was caring

Foreword

for South Vietnamese civilian casualties while managing realistic fear for her personal safety that I had never had to know. It turns out Sung, as well as I, was paid for her nursing work by the U.S. government, another lesser known aspect of the war.

How Nursing Defines Itself

From early on, Sung's character and resilience were shaped by parents of strong character and faith. Of particular significance was the influence of a devoted elder brother, whose undying devotion and vision propelled her when all else fell away. A querying mind served her well over the years. With lived experience through war, wide-ranging clinical experiences, levels of professional education, and self-reflection and personal growth, Sung Yoo is singularly qualified to contribute to the larger nursing, as well as historical, literature. "Professional identity, influenced by one's personal identity and unique background, is formed throughout one's education and career."[1]

In documenting her life story, Sung Yoo has provided not only a fascinating narrative but also an unusual exemplar of that evolution toward a professional identity. In so doing, she hopes to inspire others to consider becoming a nurse.

An American Nurses Association definition of nursing encompasses the lifespan from birth through death. "Nursing integrates the art and science of caring and focuses on the protection, promotion, and optimization of health and human functioning; the prevention of illness and injury; the facilitation of healing; and the alleviation of suffering through compassionate presence. Nursing is the diagnosis and treatment of human responses and advocacy in the care of individuals, families, groups, communities, and populations in the recognition of the connection of all humanity."[2] Given this breadth, it becomes apparent that nursing can be, and is, practiced everywhere. Indeed, one of the attractions of the field is the potential to work virtually anywhere, in a variety of settings, along with the flexibility to change.

Sung and I were both fortunate to enter nursing in the mid–20th century, just as the education of a professional nurse was shifting to collegiate rather than hospital apprentice preparation. The time was

Sung C. Yoo and the Evolution of a Professional Identity

right for development of programs leading to a baccalaureate degree in nursing, the BSN. Later, our respective master's programs opened our eyes to broader, more expansive intellectual concepts and interdisciplinary relationships that allowed us to perform more thoughtfully, more deliberatively, more effectively with patients and colleagues.

Before the 1800s, care of the ill and infirm was done by family or friends. With industrialization and urbanization in the 19th century, hospitals began to proliferate to take care of those who had no other help. Nursing care was variable. If hospitals were operated by religious nursing orders, care was of good quality. If not, care was highly uneven.[3]

During the mid–19th century, nursing began to develop into a discipline. For this, Florence Nightingale, the British nurse noted for her humanitarian work during the Crimean War (1853–56), was substantially responsible. Nursing was "both a science and an art," she thought, and nurses should focus on the "whole patient," including body, mind, and spirit. This was essential to improving the patient's health and recovery. "The concepts of health, healing, well-being, and interconnectedness with the multidimensional environment were noted in her work."[4] Not only did Nightingale's enormous impact have a key transformative effect on Sung Yoo, but it also transformed nursing and education for nurses worldwide.

Over the first half of the 20th century, hospitals took over the training of nurses in two- or three-year programs. Hospitals utilized their students as staff who provided the majority of patient care in an apprentice-like system, learning on the job, without pay, graduating with a diploma as a trained nurse. State nursing associations began organizing, influencing state nurse registration acts, providing a licensing system for nurses resulting in the title "Registered Nurse" (RN).[5]

Over the last half of the 20th century, demands increased for better educated nurses and better staffed workplaces. Dramatic advances in medicine and technology in the 1930s and during the World War II era rendered past routine patterns of practice by student caregivers insufficient. Modern intensive healthcare systems—for example, intensive care units and coronary care units—became more widespread. Safety and quality now depended on nurses' ability to utilize critical thinking and clinical judgment, to independently recognize and solve patient care problems. The expectations of both the public and nurses themselves changed.[6]

At the same time, within the profession there was debate about the best preparation. In a supposed temporary compromise, community college–based programs (also known as associate degree programs) were proposed and created "to provide technically skilled nurses to meet the immediate demand until enough baccalaureate degree nurses could be trained."[7] They remain a popular way to enter the nursing profession even today.

Yet the move to higher education was very much underway as Sung and I began our nursing studies. By 1960, there were around 172 college-based nursing programs awarding bachelor of science in nursing degrees.[8] The baccalaureate degree in nursing was the recommended route for preparation and the "way of the future" for advancement, I was told, as was Sung. Indeed, that proved true.

With the increasingly complex demands of patient care in the latter 20th century, studies were showing that educational levels mattered. Linda Aiken's rigorous research studies even demonstrated a "causal link between increased employment of BSN's and lower mortality in hospitals over time, giving hospital leaders confidence that investments in BSN's will yield value to their organizations."[9] BSNs are so valued, in fact, that many employers offer financial incentives in support of RN-to-BSN staff or, in Sung Yoo's case, to postgraduate education.

Economic Security

Early in Sung Yoo's life as a young woman, nursing was a way out of poverty. Given the devastated economy of South Korea in her early career, adequate income continued to be a concern well into her career. Finances are a concern in the United States, too. Traditionally, nursing has been an occupation for women. Reflecting the times in the United States, it was only "in the mid-twentieth century nursing abandoned its objectional system of race and gender segregation, opening up equal educational, professional, and employment opportunities."[10] Although the numbers are growing, men now make up just 12 percent of the nursing population.[11] Women's work in general is known to be less remunerative, and nurses have often felt (and actually have been) underpaid for their stressful and demanding work. Before mid-century, private duty nursing, on an ad hoc basis, was the most available job post hospital training. It was only by 1950 that salaried employment of staff nurses in hospitals became the norm.[12] Pay has always been an issue, but increased demand, professional advocacy, and levels of education and specialization have all driven pay to higher levels. Whether in times of nursing shortages or not, employment opportunities continue to be available.

Nursing, Respect, and Status

Sung's reluctance to consider nursing stemmed from a culturally induced lack of respect that she admittedly internalized. Initially, nursing felt beneath her, comparable to a maid, she explains, attributing this to her Korean cultural perspective. While the nature of direct care does necessitate contact with all manner of bodily processes and requires tasks, modern nursing care imbues even these caring tasks with much more sophistication and clinical judgment.

Interestingly, Sung's (and nursing's) deserved heroine, Florence Nightingale, "made nursing so respectable at the time that she drew well-to-do, middle-class British women into nursing."[13] Comparably, in the United States, some of the later 19th- and early 20th-century advances were made by privileged and well-educated American women such as Lillian Wald, a pioneer in the field of public health (the very arena in which Sung had her first job). Wald worked in New York where, in 1893, she established the Henry Street Settlement House which provided nursing and other social services to impoverished populations on the Lower East Side.[14] No matter the status or economic background, nursing has supported "both the class aspirations and the genuine mobility of diverse social groups."[15]

Respect for nursing has been an issue with which American nursing has also struggled. Consistently, nurses rank among the most trusted healthcare professionals, while not always the most respected.[16] Sometimes self-respect has been known to waver—for example, *"I'm only a nurse."* This issue certainly ties in with nurses' education. "While experience is always valuable in learning to recognize and intervene ... authority and expertise are almost always associated with educational attainment,"[17] writes Joan E. Lynaugh. Whereas Sung and I both sought and achieved postgraduate education, the nursing profession itself continues to discuss and aim higher in its "entry into practice" requirements at a level comparable to other professions. Currently, RN-to-BSN programs are attractive for further advancement to key clinical roles in hospitals such as clinical nurse educators and clinical nurse managers. Specialty areas, including, for example, nurse practitioners, nurse anesthetists, nurse midwives, and nurse academic educators and researchers, all require postgraduate education. For nurses, more knowledge, experience, and expertise increase self-respect as well as meet the demands of patient care.

The 1960s and '70s of our early careers were fertile times for public policy advantageous to nurses. Interestingly, our respective countries' policy initiatives at the time dovetailed to benefit both Sung and me. In the 1960s and '70s in Korea, jobs were scarce, and the Korea Overseas Development Corporation encouraged medical professionals—doctors and nurses—and others to emigrate so that their better earnings could be partially returned home and reinvested to enhance their war-weakened economy.[18] In turn, the United States, suffering severe post–World War II nursing shortages, encouraged immigration of foreign nurses to supplement the increased demands of hospitals. In 1965, the United States ended its discriminatory quota system for immigration, which opened the door for more Asian doctors and nurses as well as other professionals. Their families accompanied them upon emigration, and by 1976, 30,000 immigrants from Korea had come.[19] Sung Yoo, her husband, and their elder daughter were part of that wave in 1971.

Nursing and Cultural Adaptation

Indulgent as patients were to Sung's initial efforts to speak English, she found that working in a new language proved formidable.

Sung C. Yoo and the Evolution of a Professional Identity

Nonverbal communication plays a significant part in nursing (even different cultural norms for eye contact mattered at work), but language skills are essential. Reading and writing includes documentation of all sorts: assessments, orders, notes, and more. Understandably, all that was daunting to Sung as well as to thousands of other immigrant nurses. Relocation to a foreign country with very different norms and an inability to speak or understand the language is a staggeringly difficult situation to work through. "Although major reasons for migration are related to improved income and professional stature, these have overwhelmingly shown to erode upon relocation," write Stacey Newton, Jennifer Pillay, and Gina Higginbottom. "Cultural displacement appears to largely stem from communication and language differences, feelings of being an outsider and differences in nursing practice."[20] Another qualitative nursing research study suggests categories of psychological adjustment: relieving psychological stress, overcoming the language barrier, accepting American nursing practice, and adapting both to new styles of problem-solving strategies and interpersonal relationships. Such transitions take years, it was found, to adjust.[21] Sung Yoo's personal distress mirrors these studies.

In the 1960s, America saw enormous expansion in healthcare policy, notably the passage of Medicare and Medicaid, greatly increasing access to healthcare. Early in our careers, Sung and I both provided nursing care to more disadvantaged people in home settings thanks to this funding. Another significant initiative of the "Great Society" era, the Federal Nurse Training Act of 1964, authorized enormous funding for collegiate nursing education, expanding the growth of higher education, including baccalaureate, advanced practice, and PhD programs, into the next decades.[22] Federal support for the National Institute for Nursing Research in 1985 created a focal point for research as part of the National Institutes of Health, further advancing nursing's scientific clinical and basic research and training on issues of health and illness across the lifespan. Nurse researchers continue to build nursing's own body of evidence-based knowledge.

Nurses greatly value our ethical code, stated here by the American Nurses Association: "The nurse practices with compassion and respect for the inherent dignity, worth, and unique attributes of every person."[23] Early on, Sung acquired cross-cultural knowledge informally from life situations and later through jobs in South Korea, Vietnam, and the United States. Despite having borne the brunt of various cultural prejudices in her home country, she admits she never really shared these attitudes herself. Whether working with besieged Vietnamese, mostly poor and working-class Americans in District of Columbia public health work, or the elderly in a nursing home, she displays a spirit of curiosity and learning and a nonjudgmental attitude of compassion that is always very much in congruence with nursing's ethical code.

Among Sung's initial observations of work life in the United States was the relatively egalitarian nature of working relationships in the country. This is not to say that status differences do not exist in healthcare; from administrator to physician to nurse to assistive and support persons, they exist. Yet progressive organizational thinking (of which Sung saw a taste in her initial U.S. hospital job), as well as effective patient care, recognizes and insists on the value of every single employee. The code of ethics principles apply to relationships at work as well as those toward patients. Early in our respective careers, assistive staff had become widely utilized to expand needed nursing help with delegated tasks for which the registered nurse remains accountable. Sung's example of her working relationship with such an assistive person in the nursing home exemplifies the fundamentally important attitudes of respect, worth, and dignity vital not only to patient care but also to effective delegation.

After our distinctive Vietnam experiences, each of us found ourselves questioning just how and whether to proceed. Combining part-time employment with enriching liberal arts classes became a turning point for each of us. Years of maturity, experiences, and meeting challenges surely contribute to professional identity, but years aren't enough in themselves. What really "opened her eyes," as Sung vividly puts it, and changed her outlook was exposure to additional education—in her case, more *formal*, college-level coursework in the United States. The American Association of Colleges of Nursing emphasizes the value of a liberal education for nurses. "Through the study of the humanities, social sciences, and natural sciences, students develop the capacity to engage in socially valued work and civic leadership in society ... a broad world view."[24] Liberal studies in the humanities gave Sung fresh recognition of universal humanity in a new, more appreciative way. That led to an interest in graduate nursing studies, which further expanded her theoretical background and critical thinking. Learning about the radically groundbreaking work of the legendary nursing influential and theorist Florence Nightingale was transformative for Sung, enlarging what had been a more limited view. She discusses this at some length, including comparing and contrasting with herself and her family.

A Culmination for Sung Yoo: "How beautiful it is to be a nurse"

Our paradigms influence our behavior. Through lifelong learning, including experience, reflection, and collegiate education, Sung could embrace her role as a nurse—once chosen so reluctantly—and flourish in it. She and her story fully embody the descriptor: "Professional identity, influenced by one's personal identity and unique background, is formed throughout one's education and career. Nursing identity flourishes through engagement and reflection in multiple experiences that is defined by differing perspectives and voices. As a result, nurses embrace the history, characteristics, and values of the discipline and think, act, and feel like a nurse. Professional identity formation is not a linear process but rather one that responds to challenges and matures through professional experiences as one develops confidence as a nurse."[25] Sung Yoo has found the value of nursing for herself and ultimately elevated it for others in this extraordinary testimony. Through telling her story, the author hopes to encourage others to consider becoming a nurse. In writing these memoirs, she has achieved, for every reader, inspiration through adversity and a testimonial to the human spirit.

Lynn Hamilton *received her BSN from Washington University in St. Louis and a master's in nursing from the University of California, San Francisco. She enlisted in the U.S. Army Nurse Corps and was stationed in Yokohama, Japan, 106th General Hospital, a 1,000-bed facility entirely devoted to U.S. Vietnam War casualties. She was an educational nurse specialist for nursing staff development across the University of Michigan Hospitals and Health System for 28 years.*

Introduction

Sung C. Yoo's Place in History

by E. TAYLOR ATKINS

The Democratic People's Republic of Korea (DPRK) is probably the most successfully totalitarian regime that has ever existed (if the words "democratic," "people's," and "republic" are in the formal name of a nation-state, it's most likely authoritarian). It is the only example of a communist dynasty, ruled by three generations from one family: "Great Leader" Kim Il-sung (1912–94), "Dear Leader" Kim Jong-il (1941 or 1942–2011), and "Respected Comrade" Kim Jong-un (b. 1982, 1983, or 1984). While condemning the "feudalism" (*bonggeon jedo*) of the 518-year-old Yi royal government (1392–1910), the Kim regime has essentially reestablished hereditary monarchy in Korea.

The DPRK is the bellicose, nuclear-armed enfant terrible of East Asia, randomly firing missiles into the sea on Japan's west coast whenever it feels ignored. As I write this, news has arrived of a new "defensive" security pact, the "Treaty on Comprehensive Strategic Partnership," with Vladimir Putin's fascist Russian Federation, committing each party to provide "all means at its disposal without delay" in case the other is attacked or invaded.[1] This from two aggressively revanchist countries, one that invaded Ukraine without provocation and the other that for decades has used military force, sabotage, and covert aggression to force a political reunification of the Korean peninsula.

No wonder Sung C. Yoo's family wanted to flee North Korea. They could not have predicted how bad it would be or the severity of oppression, destitution, and starvation that awaited those who did not or

Introduction

could not leave. They only dimly understood what "communism" even meant. But they knew enough to realize they had to leave. The harrowing circumstances of their southward flight, which Ms. Yoo recounts so vividly, were temporary; for their neighbors left behind, terror and deprivation would be a permanent condition.

It's easy to forget what Russians, Chinese, Koreans, Cambodians, Cubans, Vietnamese, Angolans, and so many others found attractive about communism. Many Americans seem to think it was simply the spawn of Satan. No, it was the product of industrial capitalism, an economic system that worked well enough for some and not at all well for millions more. Communism promised the eventuality of a classless society in which both opportunity and outcome were essentially guaranteed. It was also described as an inevitable end point of human development: if history was an account of social evolution through "dialectical materialism," successive upheavals that ended one socioeconomic order and started another, then communism meant the end of history itself. However, impatient revolutionary leaders like V.I. Lenin, Mao Zedong, Fidel Castro, and Kim Il-sung were afraid the workers' revolution Karl Marx predicted wouldn't happen until after they died. So they hurried it along.

Korea's industrial revolution occurred under the yoke of Japanese imperial rule (1910–45), but the factory workforce, while growing, was far outnumbered by agricultural labor (*nongmin*). So, as Mao Zedong did in China, Kim Il-sung placed his hopes for a proletarian revolution on them. They had multiple legitimate grievances, and untold thousands of them proved receptive to the idea of seizing land from absentee landlords and Japanese imperialists, ending tenancy, eating what they grew, improving their working conditions, and otherwise taking charge of their own lives with Korean sovereignty restored.

According to Kim Il-sung, political independence without social revolution was meaningless and an undesirable delay of the inevitable. He had no interest in the prolongation of what he considered exploitative social relations, whether traditional or capitalist. After the abrupt, unanticipated liberation that accompanied Japan's surrender on August 15, 1945, he and the Workers' Party of Korea (WPK, successor to an earlier Korean Communist Party) set about the work described at the opening of Ms. Yoo's account. She tells of near-constant surveillance and harassment by WPK members trying to root out capitalists and collaborators with the Japanese regime. Like many other prosperous Koreans, Ms. Yoo's father had been both.

"Collaboration" is not a neutral word in Korean parlance. One of the harshest descriptions of the southern Republic of Korea (ROK) in DPRK propaganda is that it was from inception a nest of former collaborators (*chin'ilpa*, "pro–Japan clique," or *builbae*, "comrades attached to Japan"), an epithet that immediately calls into question the legitimacy and nationalist credentials of the southern regime. In a lecture given less than a month after liberation, Kim Il-sung made the following accusation:

> The advocates of setting up a bourgeois republic in our country are none other than comprador capitalists. They are pro–Japanese elements and traitors to the nation who, during the colonial rule of Japanese imperialism, betrayed the country and the people and worked hand in glove with the Japanese imperialists in oppressing and exploiting our people. Hardly had US troops landed in south Korea than the pro–Japanese elements and traitors to the nation advocated pro–Americanism and, with the backing of the imperialist forces, are plotting to set up a reactionary government in our country and take our people along the road to anti-democracy....
>
> At present, pro–Japanese elements and traitors to the nation are making desperate efforts to recover their old position. Alleging that our country "should be placed under mandate" they are engaged in acts of treachery that run counter to the fundamental interests of the whole nation.[2]

Kim's characterization of the southern regime as infested with collaborators was unfair in the sense that many of them had unassailable nationalist credentials. The ROK's first head of state, Syngman Rhee, was one of them. But neither was Kim's denouncement completely inaccurate. After all, so-called collaborators were the only ones who had the education, experience, and expertise necessary to build a new state and modern economy from scratch (Kim Il-sung of course rejected this notion, insisting that the emerging "people's committees" were up to the task). Nevertheless, some three or four generations after the establishment of the ROK government on August 15, 1948, the stench of collaboration still lingers as a political liability, in part because many descendants of *chin'ilpa* retain generational wealth to this day.

Defining collaborators as "those who received titles under Japanese rule, arrested or killed independence fighters," the government

Introduction

appointed a Presidential Committee for the Inspection of Collaboration for Japanese Imperialism, which initially identified around 1,000 such individuals.³ But to many, the government's definition was far too narrow: critics said it should include schoolteachers, police officers, and Koreans employed in the colonial bureaucracy, not to mention brokers who deceitfully recruited girls to work in Japanese military bases, the so-called comfort women.

In the mid–2000s, the private Institute for Research in Collaborationist Activities began investigating *chin'ilpa* and compiled public lists of thousands of names, arranged into 13 categories. "Even if they engaged in no particular pro–Japanese acts," chairman Yoon Kyoung-ro announced, "if they were in a certain position they must take social responsibility."⁴ Punishments included seizure of assets that were deemed ill-gotten through collaboration. Sheila Miyoshi Jager points out that "critics of the truth committees say the effort is politically motivated and in a society where offspring are judged guilty by family association, they maintain that the truth committees are simply attempts to damage certain politicians." However, Jager observes, the stakes are even higher as each regime jockeys for legitimacy as the representative of the Korean people everywhere: "The struggle over Korea's colonial past is really a struggle over the two Korea's [sic] future."⁵

The Korean War that shattered the peninsula and definitively shaped Ms. Yoo's life can be traced back to several possible origin points on the historical timeline. One thing that is often forgotten, however, is that it was a war between Koreans and in a formal sense is ongoing (it ended with a ceasefire). As two ideological factions coalesced as rival states in 1948, each chose a mightier champion to back its cause: the north aligned with the Soviets and the south with the Americans. Thus did a civil conflict in a small, postcolonial country become a "proxy war" in the early Cold War, involving well over 20 combatants.⁶ It's easy to blame a handful of meddling outsiders—Japan, China, the United States, the Soviet Union, and Western European imperial powers—for the conflict, and they do indeed bear some responsibility. Nonetheless, a variety of internal cleavages made some sort of eventual civil conflict among Koreans not inevitable (nothing is) but at least foreseeable.

Sung C. Yoo's Place in History

For centuries, Korean society was rigidly hierarchical and favored bloodline lineage over merit and accomplishment. Even during the Edo period (1600–1868), Japanese society, with its formalized, endogamous status system distinguishing warriors from farmers, artisans, and merchants based on the same neo–Confucian ideals to which Koreans gave allegiance, allowed some workarounds and a degree of flexibility when necessary, such as matrilocal and intercaste marriage and purchase of warrior status by wealthy commoners.

Under the Yi dynasty, four status groups were recognized: hereditary aristocrats (*yangban*); an intermediate class of educated petty bureaucrats and skilled workers (*jungin*); urban and rural commoners (*sangmin*); and a lowborn "unclean" caste (*cheonmin*). A cultural distinction can also be made between a patriarchal, Sinocentric Confucianist governing class and commoners who lived under a more gender-flexible (if not matriarchal) society in which female shamans (*mudang*) held considerable social capital. During the years of authoritarian rule in the ROK, nongoverning commoners were idealized as "the people" (*minjung*), historically a more purely "Korean" force for democracy.

Ms. Yoo's memoir also draws attention to the considerable regional differences among Koreans. Dialects were so distinct as to be mutually unintelligible. Refugees from the north encountered hostility from southerners, whom Ms. Yoo's father described as culturally backward because of their agricultural practices, among other things (the feeling was mutual: her future mother-in-law opposed her marriage because "northern women were seen as having poorer manners than southern women"). As in China, India, Italy, and the United States, there were palpable cultural differences between northern and southern cultures (as well as within them), which provided at least some basis for the geopolitical partition of the Korean peninsula.

Another noteworthy status differentiation was between women and men. Although it was hardly unique in this respect, Korean society was based on firm male dominance, especially at the upper tiers. Some Koreans boast that their society has always been more gender egalitarian because wives do not take their husbands' surnames, but there's another way to look at it. Unlike in China or Japan, wives were not entered into official family registries (*hoju*), meaning they were

Introduction

virtually outsiders. Even as mothers, women's existence was irrelevant; offspring just magically appeared. What does this have to do with the Korean War? Communists everywhere recruited women for their cause by promising absolute gender equality, capitalizing on female resentment toward the patriarchy. Whether those promises were eventually honored after the revolution or not, much female labor went into communist movements.

Wealth gaps, which appear constantly in Ms. Yoo's account, intensified resentments within Korean society. Wealth and inherited status were not always aligned. *Yangban* aristocrats who either could not pass the government civil service exam (*gwageo*) or were not eligible to even take it because they were the sons of their fathers' secondary wives or concubines, often made meager livings as teachers or lowly bureaucrats. Commoners could be wealthy. And fortunes could change. Ms. Yoo's father was wealthy but generous; his largesse enabled him to escape the WPK cadres who were coming after him. But the Yoo family lost everything.

Sung C. Yoo is forthright about how difficult it was to give up her privileged life to make matchboxes, be a maid, and tutor the bed-wetting daughter of a prosperous family. Even in her most desperate hour, she could not abandon the idea that becoming a nurse was beneath her: she thought the nursing profession was no better than being a housemaid ("Without taking time to understand what it meant to be a nurse, I simply resented nursing, considering nurses to be a helper, maid, and servant, etc."). Her account of living with her tutee Sook's family reveals how even during the Korean War and its aftermath, some families seemed to be virtually unscathed, having plenty to eat and money to buy decent clothes and go to school. Obviously, the privations of war did not affect all equally, which partially explains why even for some southerners, communism seemed attractive. Immediately after the DPRK capture of Seoul, Ms. Yoo remarks, "Class no longer existed. Everyone was suddenly and strictly equal."

The simmering resentments among Koreans were sharply exacerbated by the imposition of Japanese rule. From the early 17th until the mid–20th centuries, both countries tried to severely limit diplomatic relations with all but a small handful of other polities. Two decades after Japan was coerced to open its borders to the great powers, it

Sung C. Yoo's Place in History

forced Korea to do so as well. Japanese officials came to regard Korea as crucial to its security, as a foothold to access commerce in continental Asia and as a geographic buffer between them and potential imperialist predators, particularly czarist Russia. In the last quarter of the 19th century, Korea showed all the signs of a failing state: a factionalized court facing socioeconomic instability and external threats with a stubborn attachment to cultural and political precedents. In the era of New Imperialism (ca. 1870–1914), as huge swaths of Africa and Southeast Asia were falling under European colonial rule, Korea seemed destined to become yet another colony.

Initially, the Japanese wanted merely a friendly, competent government on the peninsula and even sponsored a failed coup attempt in 1884 to install a pro–Japanese faction at court.[7] At the turn of the century, Japan fought two wars, against China (1894–95) and Russia (1904–05), for control of the peninsula. The peace settlement in September 1905 gave Japan unchallenged control of Korea via a "protectorate" regime that left the monarchy intact but placed diplomacy and internal security in Japanese hands. When the royals proved to be uncooperative, Japanese officials removed them from power entirely and took direct control of Korea in 1910.

The protectorate treaty itself drew sharp lines between pro–Japanese collaborators and anti–Japanese nationalists. Its Korean signatories, all ministers in Emperor Gojong's government, stole the royal seal to authorize the agreement. To this day, Japanese apologists insist that Gojong's seal made the agreement legitimate under international law, while Koreans argue otherwise because the monarch refused to ratify it personally.[8] The signatories became known as the Five Eulsa Traitors (*Eulsa ojeok*), all of whom faced immediate assassination attempts.

What followed was strict martial law under a Japanese military regime that abolished the Korean-language press and ordered the teaching of Japanese as the "national language" in schools. Yet on March 1, 1919, as the Versailles Peace Conference was convening and aspiring nation-states were being created from the remnants of the German, Austro-Hungarian, and Ottoman empires, the Korean people stood up to Japanese tyranny. In a show of national unity that seems unimaginable today, millions of Koreans marched throughout the country, emboldened by a Declaration of Independence and

Introduction

shouting *"Manse!"* (Long live Korea!). A brutal Japanese crackdown ensued in which hundreds of thousands of Koreans were arrested, tortured, mutilated, murdered, or some combination thereof.

In 1921, the colonial government announced a policy of "cultural rule," which promised to govern Koreans with a lighter hand but also aimed to invest them in a permanent Japanese presence. Some Koreans—the ones later branded collaborators—benefited socially and financially by learning Japanese, attending universities in the metropole, and working for or with the regime and Japanese corporations. Many others did not.[9] Rice farmers exported the lion's share of their crop to Japan, unable to consume it themselves.[10] With varying degrees of enthusiasm and free will, thousands of Korean laborers emigrated to Japan to work in mines, factories, and other industries as cheap labor. Japanese rule also virtually wiped out the peninsula's population of Siberian tigers, which had become symbols of Korean national identity.[11]

Like Chinese and Vietnamese, after the 1917 Bolshevik revolution in Russia, Koreans discovered Marxist-Leninist thought and organized to fight both the Japanese imperialists and traditional Korean mindsets. A more moderate group of "cultural nationalist" intellectuals eschewed the violent overthrow of Japanese imperialism, seeking rather to educate and modernize the Korean people so that they would eventually be prepared for self-government.[12] Even if the Japanese left tomorrow, they believed, Koreans were unready to take their place as a viable sovereign nation in the modern world. Radical and moderate nationalists tried to form a united front organization, the Shingan'hoe, which lasted only from February 1927 to May 1931.[13] These two broad factions—and unsurprisingly, there were factions within the factions—and a government in exile in Shanghai constituted the foundation for the ideological conflict between the DPRK and ROK regimes.

As Japanese military aggression in China intensified throughout the 1930s, Koreans were increasingly coerced to contribute to the war effort. The relatively liberal "cultural rule" policies were gradually abandoned; by the end of the 1930s, hardcore assimilation directives were designed to make Japan and Korea "one body."[14] Korea was not targeted by the Allies for aerial attacks during the Pacific War, but its people were nonetheless involved in and affected by it as soldiers and labor. Japan's surrender on August 15, 1945, immediately and unexpectedly released the colony. However, Soviet and U.S. troops soon occupied the peninsula, dividing it into two administrative zones at the 38th parallel, a border that has remained mostly unchanged ever since. Then as now, two-thirds of the peninsular population resides in the south. Although there was some migration from the south to the north, an estimated 900,000 people, some 10 percent of the population north of the 38th parallel, went in the opposite direction.[15] Sung C. Yoo's family was among them.

One of the most striking passages in Ms. Yoo's memoir describes her feelings before entering Ewha University's nursing program. Utterly "helpless and hopeless," she fell into a deep depression.

> I yearned to be in my own home again, just for one day, but that was a pipe dream. Then, what was my reason to be alive? Why didn't I die during the Korean War? Who could I blame for my current situation? The more I thought, the more I found unanswered because it was impossible to know the causes. I believed it was fate.... It was inconceivable to find out reasons. Once I felt that I was lucky and thankful to be alive through all difficulties, but now I felt guilty about being alive.... I began to review the past about what and how I had lived. The reviewing was simple: to be born in North Korea and had to live through the Korean War. In my memories, I couldn't remember what our family or myself did wrong. Rather, I asked myself, should we have stayed in North Korea and not looked for democracy?

As unique as her life story may be in some respects, Ms. Yoo's feelings of being swept up by historical events beyond her control, of being sacrificed for a dimly understood "cause" such as "democracy" (I will explain the scare quotes shortly) or communism, and of indignation, homesickness, hunger, insecurity, and injustice were shared by millions of Koreans.

Koreans have a word, *han*, that can be translated as "resentment" or "indignant sorrow" and that many of them claim is a national cultural trait. Implicit in the concept is the realization that *someone* is to blame, whether predatory outside powers or corrupt, incompetent, and callous domestic political elites who cared little about the suffering their grand ambitions entailed. Ms. Yoo's early life was suffused with *han*. But she was hardly alone.

During her year-long sojourn as a nurse in war-torn Vietnam, she

Introduction

witnessed an eerily familiar situation—a conflict between "democracy" and communism fought between neighbors with backing from Cold War superpowers—and felt deep sympathy for those who suffered terror, injury, and death. The Vietnamese she met seemed more accustomed to war than Koreans had been and were able to carry on with daily life. She notes the compassion that South Vietnamese nurses showed toward Vietcong insurgents whom they had every reason to hate, contrasting this with the bitter animosity between communists and noncommunists in her homeland. But like Koreans, many of the people she met had only the dimmest idea of what this war was even about, let alone why they had to suffer so terribly for it.[16]

The fact of the matter is that relatively few Koreans and Vietnamese understood what communism was, let alone "democracy." I keep putting that latter word in scare quotes because both southern regimes (under Syngman Rhee and Park Chung-hee in the ROK and Ngo Dinh Diem in the Republic of Vietnam) were dictatorships, every bit as cruel and rigidly authoritarian as their communist foes. Both were comprised of nationalist elites who had benefited socially and economically from prior colonial regimes, and fairly or not, both were accused of being neocolonial compradors propped up by the United States. During the Cold War, the United States supported dictatorships in Latin America, Southeast Asia, Africa, and the Middle East as faux democracies so long as their leaders were staunchly anti-communist.[17] Little wonder, then, that most Koreans and Vietnamese had no clue what "democracy" was. They never experienced it.

Ms. Yoo's memoir is instructive not only about Korean experiences of partition, civil war, social divisions and prejudices, and Korean participation in the Vietnam War but also about Asian immigration to the United States and Asian American history. In 1965, a monumental change in U.S. immigration law abolished the National Origins Formula, an inherently racist quota system that had severely restricted migration from anywhere other than Western and Northern Europe for four decades.

According to the Migration Policy Institute, immigration from South Korea increased exponentially, 2,500 percent between 1965 and 1980. It nearly doubled in the 1980s and then again by 2010. Close political and military ties between the ROK and the United States have no doubt made it easier for Koreans than for other Asian immigrants to enter the United States and become naturalized citizens. Koreans are also favored because they "tend to be highly educated and of high socioeconomic standing compared to other immigrant groups and the overall U.S.–born population."[18]

Ms. Yoo was among the first wave of migrants who were welcomed to address a critical shortage of nurses.[19] For some time now, immigrant nurses have been indispensable to the U.S. medical system; it could not have functioned during the 2020 Covid pandemic without nurses from the Philippines.[20]

Ms. Yoo repeatedly says that the single most daunting hurdle she and other immigrant nurses faced was mastering the English language. It is unquestionably vital that health practitioners be able to communicate clearly with their patients. Beyond learning conversational English, they must master the terminology and conventions of medical communication. During the time that Ms. Yoo was learning and teaching nursing, it seems that many immigrant nurses were not receiving adequate language training before coming to the United States.

Most Americans have never studied another language and have no appreciation for how difficult English is, let alone compassion or patience for those struggling to learn it. English speaking has become a major "culture war" issue. Some municipalities have tried to make English their official, mandatory language for conducting business, refusing to staff offices or schools with bilinguals, while posting signs (often with incorrect spelling and punctuation) to reinforce the point.[21] Some Americans scream at people they hear speaking another language in public spaces. Since Asian immigrants, in particular, have faced harsh discrimination for speaking English with noticeable accents, many parents have decided it's best not to let their children learn their heritage tongue.[22]

Ms. Yoo does not describe any such prejudice, nor do we learn if she and her husband taught their three children Korean. But she does indicate how critical it was for nurses to master English for their education and communication with patients. It is interesting that in her account, the first Korean students she taught at Eastern University in 2005 do not seem to have been any better prepared linguistically than

Introduction

she was in the 1960s and 1970s. Considering that English is a mandatory subject in Korean public schools from kindergarten and that around 30,000 U.S. troops are based in the ROK, some with their families, this is somewhat surprising.[23] However, one of the long-standing criticisms of English-language education in the ROK and Japan is that conversation is downplayed in a curriculum focused on grammar and vocabulary "taught to the test," with the eventual aim of passing university entrance exams. It might be fair to say that English is taught as if it were mathematics.

Ms. Yoo explains in great detail the culture shock she experienced after arriving in the United States. It is an experience common to immigrants everywhere, but she lays out plainly the challenges of adapting to entirely different modes of social interaction. In her case, she found the change refreshing. She describes how every conversation in the Korean language signals differences in status between the participants: there are entirely different pronouns and verb conjugations for speaking with someone older or younger, of different rank or status, classmates in different grade levels, or for the gender of the speakers. It is not true that American English has no such distinctions whatsoever—we don't speak to our bosses, strangers, or parents exactly the same way as to our friends or siblings—but Ms. Yoo finds English to be less ritualized or formal in general, acknowledging a greater degree of equality between people than she was accustomed to.

She also notes differences in classroom interactions and pedagogy. Having taught many international students, I can testify personally that an interactive, conversational classroom in which student input is incorporated, valued, and considered a best practice is quite alien to most of them (this is not true only of East Asians; many students from Europe also are more accustomed to deferential, teacher-focused, "sage on the stage" pedagogy). As an educator and mentor to Korean immigrant nurses, Ms. Yoo encountered student reticence to think critically and creatively about their subject matter. But she did so from a position of sympathy and understanding rather than frustration because she had had to learn to overcome her own inhibitions as she continued her own education and professional development.

Sung C. Yoo's Place in History

She frequently mentions Confucianism as the core of Korean ethics and social relations and as a key inhibitor of intellectual independence and social equality. Although it is true that the Chinese philosopher Confucius taught the naturalness of hierarchy in social relations and believed that social harmony could best be attained through ritualized observance of filial piety (*xiao,* reverence for one's parents and ancestors), I maintain that Confucius considered *reciprocity* to be the core for differential social relations. That is, his teachings emphasize the inherent dignity and perfectibility of *all* humans. Social authority was based not on inborn nobility but on accomplishment, self-cultivation, and self-mastery.

As his most important intellectual descendant Mencius explained, one was worthy of deference only to the extent that one showed wisdom, benevolence, compassion, mercy, and empathy to those of lower rank. Parents must show genuine care for their children and respect their dignity as human beings. Rulers must look after and prioritize the welfare of their subjects; otherwise, they were not worthy of being rulers. Mencius insisted that loyalty and submission were conditional, not absolute, and that those in authority are accountable for the well-being of the people under their care.[24]

Unfortunately, in practice Confucianism became justification for demanding absolute obedience to parental or political authority, regardless of how the person of higher rank behaved. Ms. Yoo grew up within a context in which Confucianism meant unquestioned submissiveness to precedent and authority. This carried over into education as well. Education meant rote mastery of long-standing bodies of knowledge handed down over generations by wise sages, which were not to be challenged. The irony is that a quotation attributed to Confucius in the *Analects* is a plain endorsement of critical thinking and intellectual independence: "Learning without thought is labor lost; thought without learning is perilous."[25]

Translated to Ms. Yoo's field, "learning" in nursing would be the technical medical knowledge required in the profession; "thought" would obviously be critical thinking or what she calls "nursing theory," the conceptual foundations for the profession that she attributes to Florence Nightingale. For her, Confucianism was the basis for her own initial and long-held notion that nurses were merely "housemaids" and

Introduction

servants to elite physicians. It is unfortunate that in her experience Confucianism was primarily an oppressive, anti-intellectual hurdle and cultural handicap that Korean nurses must overcome to prosper in the United States.

Be that as it may, Sung C. Yoo made it her life's mission to elevate the profession in Korean society. Her advocacy of nursing as a noble calling surely had an impact on the self-regard of later generations of Korean immigrant nurses and, by extension, contributed to the health and welfare of thousands of patients.

I was asked to write this introduction because, although my primary field of expertise is Japanese history, I have researched, written, and taught extensively about modern Korean history as well. My charge was to provide historical context for Ms. Yoo's memoir. Reading it brought to mind many other firsthand accounts and scholarship I have read over the last quarter of a century. There are many possible historical threads to pull together, and if someone else had written this, it might look substantially different. I believe that future scholars working on the history of the nursing profession, immigration, Asian America, women's history, and politics, culture, and society in post-liberation Korea will find *From North Korea to America Through Three Wars* to be instructive and illuminating.

However, I will not pretend to have read Sung C. Yoo's autobiography with only a historian's eyes. It is enlightening in a spiritual way as well. Spirituality need not involve religion; at its core, it is recognition that something exists outside our individual selves, that we are connected to and have ethical obligations to the world in which we live and the people with whom we share it, whether we know them or not. Ms. Yoo is an avowed Christian and I a Baha'i, yet I can identify with her periodic crises of faith, which are less an indication of spiritual weakness than a sign that we are paying attention to our own feelings and those of others, to injustice, ignorance, and unnecessary suffering caused by human decisions *not* informed by spirituality as defined above.

We do not all endure the degree of material privations and psychological misery that Ms. Yoo and millions of other Koreans did under colonial rule, the sudden restoration of sovereignty, partition and family separation, and the Korean War. The people who, for whatever reason, did not achieve the sense of fulfillment that she did were not failures. Many, perhaps most, of them showed the same "bootstrapping" grit and determination, yet did not prosper as she did. I can't explain why, nor should we heed anyone who pretends to know.

What we need to ask ourselves, then, is what do we do with the success, luck, or blessings (however one wishes to couch it) that we receive but that others inexplicably don't? How can we create a world in which *more* people who endure unspeakable suffering can prosper?

Ms. Yoo shows us: she uses her experience to serve humanity, as a healer, teacher, role model, and possessor of wisdom. When she asks her Korean nursing students, "See what I did. Why can't you do it?" she is not just urging them to buy into the American bootstrap ideology of pursuing individual economic prosperity and social recognition. She is also asking if they, too, can and will use what they learn to benefit *everyone* whom they nurse, to use their own pain to alleviate that of others.

E. Taylor Atkins *is Distinguished Teaching Professor of history at Northern Illinois University. His publications include* Kogun by the Toshiko Akiyoshi-Lew Tabackin Big Band *(2024);* A History of Popular Culture in Japan, From the Seventeenth Century to the Present *(2017; second edition, 2022);* Primitive Selves: Koreana in the Japanese Colonial Gaze, 1910–1945 *(2010);* Jazz Planet *(2003); and* Blue Nippon: Authenticating Jazz in Japan *(2001).*

Prologue
An Unexpected Moment

It was my first day at Eastern University in Pennsylvania, and although I was extremely nervous, I was honored to be working as an adviser in the Department of Nursing's RN-to-BSN program for Korean nurses. I was eager to work with these students because I, too, am a Korean nurse who moved to America. But unlike these nurses, I had recently learned the value of nursing, overcoming cultural prejudices against the profession. In Korea where I was born, nursing was seen as a lowly occupation. I never wanted to be a nurse; however, I never expected my life to turn out how it did. It took a lifetime of struggles through three wars, poverty, depression, and the pain of leaving my family behind, but with words of encouragement from my brother, Sung Kul, who told me to never quit, I now appreciate and love being a nurse. This is the story of how I overcame poverty and survived through three wars to become a nurse. I thank God for guiding me to this career, and I want to share my story with other nurses, especially future nurses, so that they can see how beautiful it is to be a nurse and appreciate all that they will do for the whole world, just like Florence Nightingale said. This is an exciting moment I thought I could not have in life. But here it is; it came.

Prologue

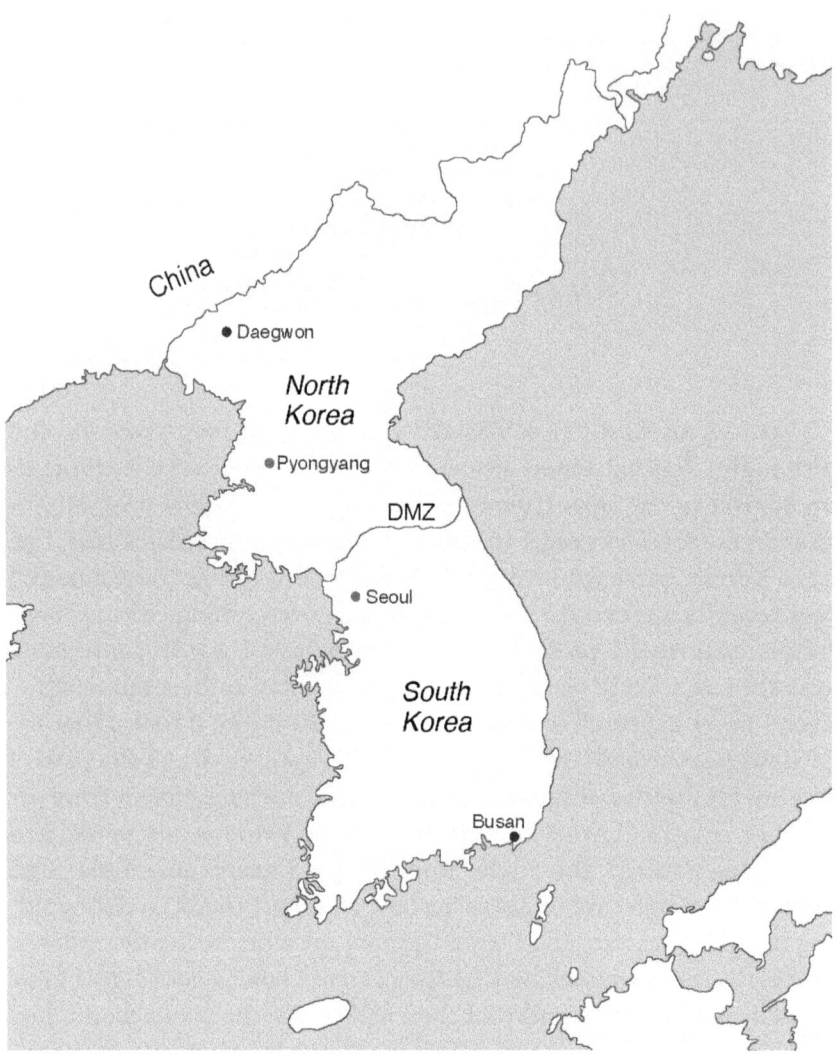

Map of Korea, courtesy Clyde H. Mapping, under license https://creativecommons.org/licenses/by-sa/4.0/deed.en, Wikimedia Commons. Modified (all wording) by Tisha S. Woo.

I

Leaving North Korea

One morning when I woke up, my mother, Tae Won Kim, told me, "If anyone asks where your father is, answer 'I absolutely do not know.'" I was eight years old at that time and living at 228 Daegwon-dong, Oenam-myeon, Sagju-gun, Pyonganbuk-do in what is now North Korea.

My hometown was located not far from the border between northern Korea and China. It was a small town with only one elementary school and one high school and no college. Also, there was only one church. That was the reason why almost everyone knew everybody. Every five days, there was a market where everyone gathered their wagons or cows to sell merchandise in the cold weather; this far up north, it was often colder than the U.S. state of Maine. In winter, children used to ice skate easily anywhere, but they could swim in the summer when it was clement. The trees in all green resembling Canada were tight and close in high mountains. The water was potable anywhere; while walking or hiking, there was no need to be cautious. In Korea, the nature was very pure at that time. The Japanese enjoyed this nature very much while they occupied Korea for 36 years until 1945.

Born in 1892, my father, Yuen Kuen Lee, was a well-known businessman. During World War II, he owned Samil Enterprise Co., Ltd. (삼일 기업주식회사), along with a Joseon soy sauce shipping company and a local timber business. This was when cars were not widely available and most people used wagons, so his shipping businesses were very profitable. At that time, many Koreans were hungry because the Japanese government was responsible for rationing and distributing rice, soybeans, grains, etc., to the Korean people. In this system, food was rare, but our family was not struggling because my father had enough grains from his business. Fortunately, the Japanese treated my father with respect because of his businesses. He and my mother used to share our food with many neighbors. He owned all the land in the town and had provided the land for the school, the township, and the church that he used to attend every day for early morning prayer.

    In 1910, my father was the first person in my hometown to convert to Christianity, thanks to an American missionary, Henry Willard Lampe. Every month, the missionary visited Daegwon-dong, riding his motorcycle to my hometown from Sunchon, where he lived with his wife. Everyone in town eagerly awaited his visit not because they wanted to become Christian, but to see his motorcycle, which was new to us in Daegwon-dong, and his American face. It was the first time the townspeople saw an American. When my father met Lampe, he became a believer in Jesus. He immediately embraced the teachings of Christ; in fact, he remained devoted to Jesus until he died while a refugee in Mogpo in 1951. When he learned about Jesus from Lampe, my father incinerated the rice-straw idols of Korean deities in our house in a firepit outside. Shocked by my father's actions, my mother feared she would lose a child for his heresy, but the next day, all her children were still healthy and alive. She was relieved. Every morning at 4:00 a.m., he exercised in his bed and then headed to church, waking up the neighborhood women along the way by coughing when he passed by their homes. Back then, not many people owned a watch and clock, and waking up on time during the cold winter was arduous, so my father's coughing served as an alarm to wake them up to make a fire, warm water for cleaning, and prepare breakfast for their families. He was stern and kept firm when it came to being on time. His eagerness for education was extremely high. He was self-made and self-taught, which earned him admiration and trust from our village. He taught my mother the Korean alphabet (Hangul) using the sandbox instead of paper because my mother was totally illiterate. They used an oil lamp since there was no electricity. Finally, she reached the level where she could read the Bible with some difficulty. He directed my mother to follow the weekly menu, according to his calculations of nutrition, to make sure we were well fed. Since my mother was not educated, she was unable to understand why he made a weekly menu, which was restricted in many ways. She often had a hard time because she was not able to relate with nutrition at all back then.

My mother gave birth to ten children, but only five of us survived, three boys and two girls, including me. I was the ninth of ten children. My oldest brother, Sung Hee, was already grown up, and my older sister Sung Sook was married when I was in first grade. My second oldest brother, Sung Kul, was in middle school, and my baby brother, Sung Duk, was two years younger than me. My house chores included cleaning the thin glass lamp that we used at night because there was no electricity. It was very fragile and easily breakable, so I had to be careful when wiping off the smoke residue. Often, I would accidentally break the glass when cleaning the lamp. My father recorded these mistakes in a notebook; he had notebooks for each child. The third time it happened, my father punished me by hitting me on the palms and calves with the strong stick that he kept above the doorframe. If I moved or cried, I got more hits from my father. Right after he hit me, he showed me how I had made a mistake and explained why I was being punished. Although I was under strict instructions from my father, I used to make that kind of mistake often because the glasses were so thin and delicate. My mother would help me, so I would not make the mistake again. I never appreciated this chore, and I was afraid of my father; I didn't understand his strict parenting style. When he was away on business trips, I was happy as could be because there were no rules or chores. As I got older, I realized that my father was the best teacher for me. I greatly appreciated and admired him after his death.

I went to first grade at the elementary school built on the land donated by my father. Everyone, of course, knew about me and who I was because of the name of my father. Not only that, but I was vivacious and active, with many friends in school. In no way was I a traditional girl of that era. My father often said that he wished that I had been born as a boy. At that time, I did not understand why he said that, but my mother laughed. Because I was a girl, my father said that I should be calm and quiet, and although he tried to treat all his children equally, he discriminated between his sons and daughters.

Nevertheless, I took a leader's position in the class. Every fall, the school held an athletic meet, and at the end, there was a marathon between Cheong-gun (blue team) and Hong-gun (red team). I was the first runner because I was a first grader. Over the last decade, Hong-gun had always won, but not in that year because I ran faster from the beginning than the other team. My older brothers and others threw me in the air like a ball to celebrate. That moment I could never forget. The band was the loudest it could be! The people shouted, chanting my name so much that their throats ruptured.

My prize for winning the race was a dozen pencils, which my father kept, and he only permitted me to use one. He wanted to teach me to be thrifty, but I was disappointed because he was so strict and those pencils were mine. I regretted winning a prize. Had I not won anything, I wouldn't be so upset. This memory is still as fresh as a vegetable. But now, I respect what he tried to teach me even if it took me a long time.

After World War II, the Japanese left in August 1945, and Korea was divided: North Korea became communist and South Korea became democratic. At that time, I was in the first grade in elementary school, and I had to speak Japanese in the class with a Japanese name. Under Japanese occupation, Korean students were not allowed to speak Korean in the class at all. If we did for any reason, we used to get hit on the top of the head until it bled. Therefore, we, all Korean students, were afraid of the Japanese teacher to avoid being hit. Learning Japanese was the most important thing back then: calling each other Japanese names and pretending to be Japanese. So when a child cried for any reason, the parents usually said that there were Japanese police coming: "Stop crying immediately." That worked because of Japanese police's reputation. In general, we were educated to believe that Japanese people were superior to Koreans who were seen as illiterate and dirty people. With this education, we all were afraid and scared of being checked by the Japanese.

After World War II, we immediately switched back to Korean language in class with Korean names. It was the first significant change of things. At the same time, we learned the Korean alphabet (Hangul) and the Korean national anthem and the Korean flag, which was difficult to understand after living under occupation. I had never seen it before. In addition, I was told that we had "freedom" from the Japanese. That freedom word meant we no longer had to fear the Japanese

I—Leaving North Korea

police who used to be the most supreme power to all Koreans, adults and children. After liberation from Japan, we, Koreans, were free and no longer had to see the Japanese anymore. This freedom word was new and very strange to me at that time because I had never known what it really meant.

Then, politically, the Communist Party took power. The communists were searching for prominent figures to detain as they moved toward a dictatorship of the proletariat—essentially, wealthy men—across North Korea to arrest because the communists believed that no one should own private property. Being that my father owned land and was a successful businessman, he was chosen to be arrested as their first target in Daegwon-dong. One night in January 1946, the communists held a meeting solely about my father and planned to arrest him. Fortunately, his benevolence and good deeds ended up saving his life. Immediately after the communists' secret meeting, one of our neighbors who attended the meeting ran to tell my father, who was already in bed, that he was going to be arrested and sent to a camp. My father sprang out of bed and left home, telling only my mother that he was fleeing. The next morning, the communists arrived early, searching for my father, as our neighbor had warned.

I was eight years old when my mother told me not to say a word about my father. She did not need to worry; I did not know where he was or why he left. I did not even know what a communist was and why they were in North Korea. After he vanished, the secret police constantly searched our house to find any information on his whereabouts. They put red stickers on all our furniture, which meant those things were no longer ours. We were only allowed to use daily-use items, such as utensils. Sensing that I was under constant watch everywhere, including at school, on the street, or at the playground, I knew not to say a word about him to anyone, especially my friends. It was not easy to "not say a word" to close friends about my father because I used to tell them everything, but I had to keep quiet. It was no longer fun to play with friends. By the age of ten, I'd grown up quickly and very cautiously and uncomfortably, and I was even scared because I was being watched. As a result, my family and I knew that we could no longer remain in communist North Korea. Therefore, my remaining family and I, nine of us total, planned to leave for South Korea.

From North Korea to America Through Three Wars

Knowing that this would not be an easy feat, we had to be brave and determined because we had no choice. It was so sad that we had to leave our friends, family, and homeland. This decision was difficult, but it was necessary for our survival. Although we believed that South Korea would be our only chance for survival, we did not have any information to help us in our journey. We did not even know if my father was alive or dead after he left, but we hoped to ultimately be reunited with him in South Korea. We also had faith that God would guide us safely to the south. It was like reaching out to the sky with my short arms, but it was our only hope.

Never had my family needed to rely on our faith. We'd always assumed that there was a God, but this time, we had to believe. As quickly as possible, my mother carefully arranged for us to cross over the 38th parallel, presently called the demilitarized zone (DMZ). The border line is 151 miles (240 km) long and approximately 2.5 miles (4 km) wide. This zone has not been open to civilians since the Armistice in July 1953. Since then, no human footsteps have been allowed in the DMZ; only animals are permitted to cross. The division has remained between North Korea and South Korea since World War II ended.

Each of my family members moved separately to South Korea. I did not know who would be leaving and when—they simply disappeared. Day and night, the children of my family, me included, kept our plan to escape a secret. My older brothers, aged 20 and 15 at the time, escaped separately to South Korea, and I do not remember at all when they left. The last group to leave for South Korea consisted of my mother, my younger brother, Sung Duk, and me. Because my family members couldn't reveal our individual escape plans, this was the first time in my life we had to keep secrets from one another; it was intense and uncomfortable, and I was scared because no one could tell us what was going to happen if we did not escape. Being so young, I had no knowledge about what to do. I had to follow whatever happened. It was deeply confusing. At school, I was the president of my third-grade class, and at weekly educational assemblies, I had to chant, "Kim Il Sung for eternity. Overthrow Syngman Rhee" (Syngman Rhee was the first president of South Korea). I was locked in a deep dilemma: to do or not to do, and I did not have anyone to comfort me or give me advice at all. There was no other helper except my mother, who

I—Leaving North Korea

was so innocent and tender, unable to analyze news or politics, not even really knowing the meaning of communism or democracy. I had no time to be sad or to complain about being in this circumstance because I was always under surveillance by everyone's eyes. I could be caught by a teacher, classmate, or friend and taken away from my family members. It was impossible to imagine what was going to happen if I were caught. I just had to keep quiet, helpless, pretending I did not have any worries or difficulties. In the meantime, I often heard that if we were caught by the North Korean army while crossing over the DMZ, we would be killed. I felt that I was walking on the eggshells. But we had to go.

My hometown was far from the DMZ, near to the Ap Lok (Yalu) River, which is the borderline between China (Manchuria) and North Korea. In the spring of 1948, my mother told me we were going to visit an old neighbor in Pyongyang, the current capital of North Korea. I did not know that we were going to South Korea. She did so intentionally for our safety in case I might have accidently said something to my friends. I told my friends I would be away for a while, unaware that I would never return home. With my mother's elaborate plan unfolding, we arrived by train in Pyongyang for a few nights, and I didn't yet know that the city was not our destination. The city was famous in Korean history for a long time, with its very different architectures, wide roads, and historical places. It was hugely different than my hometown. Now it is the capital in North Korea. While I was there, I had a chance to visit Moranbong (모란봉), a well-known hill in Korea that looked like a giant peony blossom due to the abundance of these flowers that grew all over. I had the opportunity to open my eyes to see many things like the old Korean historical buildings, breathtaking views, and rivers, which were impossible to see in my hometown. Significantly, when I was walking around, I heard the song "Home, Sweet Home" by Sir Henry Rowley Bishop being soothingly performed by Pyongyang high school girls. That memory is still alive and fresh and a tearful kick to my heart. Even today, I'm still impressed by first seeing these high school girls in their uniforms with their black hair braided. Even now, I reminisce on these feelings, thinking how wonderful music moves human minds. I was excited to see the wide roads full of automobiles and electric cars, and boats on the Taedong River, as well as the Russian female soldiers, who wore their uniforms with black leather boots that extended up to their knees. I was fascinated by their appearances, their blond hair, faces with big eyes, and white skin. It was the first time I'd seen a woman from the West.

While I was excited and fascinated to see and hear the unexpected things that I was unable to see or imagine in my hometown, my mother learned a detailed plan of how to cross over the DMZ from the neighbor we were visiting, who was so close with our family in the past at Daegwon-dong. I do not remember all the details, but with our old neighbor's guidance, we took a train to Haeju City in Hwanghae-do because that place was close to the DMZ.

After hiding out in Haeju City for a few days, one evening at sundown, my mother told me that we had to walk all night long with a guide, who would lead us to South Korea. I do not remember how my mother arranged this guide for us, but as we expected, this middle-aged man showed up to lead us to South Korea. I had a sweater, warm enough clothes for the early spring night, and the sweater had two pockets for hard taffy (traditional rice candies that were extremely popular) that I could quickly eat to suppress coughing because I was not supposed to make any noise. I needed to make sure my mouth or throat didn't get dry because we were walking the line between life and death. The guide gave us firm instructions that we must walk non-stop to follow him until he stopped. The guide demanded that I hold on tight to my mother's skirt and not to lose my mother because there was no way to find me if things happened, and so always walk next to her. My mother had a bag on her head, which was full of clothes and South Korean money, items purely meant for our survival. We had neither food nor heavy materials on us. The guide carried Sung Duk on his back all the way through because he was too young for that long walk. It was getting dark, the moon very thin like a girl's eye line in the sky, and the guide started to walk. We all became quiet with closed mouths. My eyes were focused on my mother, and I was holding on to her skirt without knowing where to go. Our fate totally depended on this guide. At that time, I was really scared and feared something bad would happen, but I trusted my mother because she was my only hope.

Since I was solely focused on walking and following my mother, I do not remember how far we had walked, but I felt some obstacle by

I—Leaving North Korea

my feet, which was impossible to see and recognize. Suddenly, I almost fell. My mother swiftly grabbed me with her hands. The guide stopped us for a short time to figure out whether I set off an alarm or warning. Of course, muted, he waited for a while to sense for a response until he continued to walk. We walked for what felt like an impossibly long time—we didn't have a watch—but I was able to vaguely make out rice paddies with water looking like a lake. Still, we kept walking until he stopped us. Finally, I was able to see a ridge between the rice paddies. The guide instructed my mother how far and where to go to see the American and Korean armies. Also, he explained why we had to stop for a moment after I almost fell: I had tripped on a straw rope marking the border between North and South Korea. (At that time, the border was not yet permanent like it is now.) If I'd touched the rope hard, then the North Korean army would've received an alert that there were trespassers. We would've been caught. He said that we were lucky to not have been caught by them because I wasn't big enough to trigger the alert. We all felt relieved. It was then that my mother paid him—I did not know how much it was—but he thanked my mother and then left back toward Haeju City.

It was dawn and we were not yet able to see clearly. As the guide had instructed, we walked ahead for a while. The sky slowly brightened, the sun rising, and we could see rice paddies in water like what I used to see in North Korea; my surroundings looked the same as they were back home in North Korea. At that moment, I wondered why we had to walk all night long, between life and death, in the same lands. But I was told that it was due to the politics: communism and democracy. It was simply scary and terrifying. It was too much for me at that young age. My sufferings, experiences, and endurances were too heavy for me; I never had to find inner strength like this before.

There were enormous reasons for my suffering, but I had no way to know them because I was a child. I couldn't figure out what it was all about it. Weakly, I had to pretend that I had no feelings about how I used to live with my family. With confusion but no choice or explanation or support, I was pushed into the situation where I had to go on with no complaints or questions. The reason for all these agonies was simple: I was born in North Korea. I had no control over where I was born. Where could I send my blame or my questions? Into the air?

From North Korea to America Through Three Wars

I learned that I could ask the question, but the answer was not there because it was too complicated and complex.

Soon we saw an American soldier and a South Korean soldier, both of whom were waving to us, signaling "Welcome." The American soldier greeted us in Korean with a funny accent, but his attitude and expression clarified what he meant. Despite our exhaustion, we laughed at his pronunciation. He reminded me of the Russian soldier in North Korea, who was tall with a big nose and white skin and wearing a green army uniform. But this American soldier wore a helmet marked "MP" in English. He was smiling at us, standing alongside the South Korean soldier, who was shorter and smaller than his American counterpart. They led us to the tent in Jangdan, Gyeonggi-do (now in North Korea), while the South Korean soldier asked my mother where we were from in North Korea. He guided us to a tent that was dark green like the army's uniforms, helmets, and cars. It had an overwhelming chemical smell. Inside, the soldier introduced us to the people who came before us. There were already many refugees from towns such as Pyongannam-do and Pyonganbuk-do in North Korea, men and women with children like me. The refugees were crammed into the tent, speaking in the heavy northern dialect. It was all so strange to me—there were so many others like us who had fled North Korea, and I had no idea. They were so delighted to see us because we had not been caught by the communists. Despite the refugees being from all different cities and towns, they had become one big family and made us feel at home. But there was no room left in the tent, no space to breathe. We slept body to body, young and old, man and woman, taking any inch of free space that we could find. Being in the tent among all these people made me realize that I immediately was no longer home in Daegwon-dong with my friends and house.

I was starving and asked my mother for food, but the refugee camp did not offer the foods that my mother used to cook. I had only ever eaten my mother's cooking because there was no fast food or junk food. But at the refugee camp, only the American's rations—dried egg, milk powder, and slim and lengthy grains—were available, which I did not want to eat because that rice was tasteless. I had never drunk milk before, and I thought that it was disgusting. The milk powder had a weird taste, almost like infant formula. Jokingly, we used to

I—Leaving North Korea

question how people could drink milk from a cow. Beyond the tent, in the nearby village, the people ate and sold the foods I was used to, so I begged my mother, who had little money to spare, to buy us something to eat. Sometimes she would say yes, but most times, she told us to eat the rations.

I began to feel even more homesick, even as I was listening to everyone saying how lucky we were that we had escaped communism. My feelings were not the same as the other refugees because my hometown had always been so comfortable and sweet, although we were under the watch of the secret police. There was no comparison between the tent and my home. The other northerners sang the hymn "The Trusting Heart to Jesus" in celebration that we would be fine in South Korea. Yes, we were free, but I felt like I was not. The food was awful. I was hungry for not only a homemade meal but also the life that I used to have at Daegwon-dong. We were safe in the tent, and I no longer had to stay quiet for fear of death, but I still missed all the good memories with friends from home. There was no comparison.

II

The Forgotten War in South Korea

After several days at the refugee camp in Jangdan, which is now part of North Korea, all the refugees, my mother, brother, and I traveled to Seoul by train to live in a center run by the Korean government. The other refugees were in high hopes on the train, singing hymns and celebrating their freedom from Kim Il-sung despite knowing nothing of politics or where exactly they would be living. Before we arrived in Seoul, the train stopped in Gaeseong City, which used to be the capital during the Joseon dynasty and is best known for ginseng tea. Some of us refugees were assigned a Jeoksan Gaok (which in Korean literally means "enemy-owned property"), usually traditional Japanese-style houses constructed during the Japanese colonial period. Clustered together with five other North Korean families, my family was placed in a serene Jeoksan Gaok, a former Japanese-occupied Buddhist temple on the side of Inwang Mountain. Other families were put up in hospitals or tents.

I do not remember how my family was assigned to this place, nor do I recall how we were reunited with my father and younger brother, Sung Kul, who crossed the DMZ on his own at 15 years old, in Seoul. We all escaped from North Korea at different times, hoping we would see one another again. One way all North Korean refugees used to meet our people was through Yeongnak Church, where North Koreans would reconnect with family members who had fled from the communists. This was the only way that we were able to meet family after we escaped from North Korea. At the end of every Sunday service, there were two types of people: those who were finally once again united with their family members and those who were sad because they did not find theirs. I was thankful to have a home in the temple, but I still did not understand why we'd fled to South Korea. I missed my friends dearly; I wished to return to Daegwon-dong to tell them all my stories, the good and bad, so we could be sad and then laugh together. At night, I used to have dreams about seeing my friends again. When I woke up, I was so disappointed because I wanted to spend more time with friends. I had these dreams up until I was 40 years old; even when I had new friends, I still had the deep experience of missing my first friends, who represented my hometown. I felt these feelings especially at sundown, watching the orange and pink sky and the bright moonlight that reminded me of Daegwon-dong. It's not easy to forget these memories.

Nevertheless, I was thankful to finally be with my family under one roof, not housed in the smelly army tent or separated. This was what we'd desperately desired under the secret watches at home in North Korea. The temple was only for sleeping, however, and all the families, including my own, had to set up a kitchen outside, exposed to the elements. We had to cook outside, no matter the weather, temperature, or season. The temple was very inappropriate for refugees because each single family needed its own kitchen and bathroom like in an apartment, but the temple was for people like us, and we had no choice at all. My mother had complained again of the reasons why we had to go through all these difficulties because Kim Il-sung took all our properties for his own benefit. Our room was only big enough for two-and-a-half tatamis, each tatami comparable to a twin-sized mattress; all five of us had to sleep, eat, and work in this room, which didn't even have a bathroom. My father built a primitive bathroom outside for all of us.

Daily life in our new city was almost impossible to compare to our life back in the north, but every family lived in these poor conditions. We felt that this was the place we were able to have freedom and our place to have our dream of a new life. Rather than complain, we had to be thankful because we were alive, trying to no longer think about or remember the past. Suddenly, I had to fit into this new environment. The temple became a typical small North Korean dwelling, all of us speaking in the same strong and heavy northern dialect, talking loudly, eating the cheap, rationed foods, and wearing worn-out and outdated clothes. We, the North Korean refugees, looked almost like beggars because we depended on rations. Despite having one another, we were discriminated against by the people in Seoul, not only because we lived like this, but because we ate and spoke differently. The southern Koreans thought we were cultureless and poor. I'd never experienced animosity like this before. We were the same people, of the same historical background, the same ancestors, yet the southerners treated us like outcasts only because of geography. The discrimination seemed natural at that time, which made me so angry, and it still exists in places in South Korea today, although it's less aggressive. Now I know that discrimination between the same people happens often during civil wars, not only in Korea.

Despite war dividing my homeland in half, the concept of class remained deeply ingrained in both northern and southern Korean culture, which originated from Confucianism. Confucianism is a philosophy and belief from China dealing with social value and culture, including morality, ethics, class, and gender. My family was once well known and respected, and we enjoyed many luxuries in life, but in South Korea, we were pariahs because we were refugees, barely scraping by. I was not welcomed to play with the South Korean girls who lived near our temple house; after all, they did not want to play with me anyway. That was surprising to me and never would have happened at home. That feeling hit me and hurt my heart; it was so sad and unforgettable. I began to ponder about the causes behind the discrimination, even Confucianism. My questions never really found answers. As such, I resented South Korean culture, and it took until recently for me to fully understand it. Even my teenage years in Seoul were as different as night and day from my life at home, where I grew up.

My father astutely observed the differences between northerners and southerners, which helped me to understand more about the southerners and why they didn't like us. He felt that southern Koreans were very much behind northerners, especially when it came to fertilizing farmlands. In the north, we mixed human feces, ashes, and plants for fertilizer, whereas southerners used only human feces. Their fertilizer often resulted in vegetable-borne diseases. When I grew up and became a nurse, I saw many South Koreans who were sick with such illnesses. According to my father, their way of farming originated from China. In his opinion, we northerners were much more advanced.

Also back then, teenage girls in South Korea were not allowed to associate with men. They couldn't look people in the eyes because they had to hide from men as women, and they weren't really allowed to be outside the home. Overall, they had to keep their distance from men outside their family. My father deplored this because he believed that teenage girls should be allowed to work.

My father always told us to never feel inferior to South Koreans because they were 30 years behind us northerners. This statement from my father made me realize that North Koreans were more practical and open-minded. The southerners were too strongly focused on what my father explained to me as the class concept of *yangban* (the aristocratic class). The *yangban* class only cared about appearances, not practicality.

One day, my father took me to a match factory to help my family, but I could not work because I didn't want to become a factory girl, which was looked down on by the people. I could not accept my lower-class status at that age. I cried and cried, unable to work all day, and I was fired by the owner of the factory. Then my father made me work from home. Along with my family members, Sung Kul, Sung Duk, and my mother, I put together matchboxes, which my father then delivered to the factory.

It was much better to work at home than in a factory, which I had never thought of in my life at that time, being from a once high-class family. But we'd become the lowest family class, and the southern girls refused to acknowledge me. Being at the factory made me feel more desperate, sad, and depressed than when I was crossing the 38th parallel. We all felt that this was a home factory and hoped things would get better. Finally, we were ready to start going to school in the spring of 1950. I enrolled in fourth grade at Taepyeongyang Elementary School, near Seoul City Hall (which no longer exists today). Before I started this school, I had severe malaria. Taking the medication quinine for malaria, my face and eyes turned yellow, but my physical condition was active, and I moved around with no problem. For this reason, again the girls at school did not want to play with me. It was another hurt. That was not my fault at all, but I felt it was. As time went by,

From North Korea to America Through Three Wars

I recovered, and my skin color returned to normal. The girls finally wanted to play with me as I'd hoped.

By this time, thanks to all my family's hard work, my father felt that we were ready to buy a house near Anguk-dong, from which many highly well-known scholars came and many *yangban* (known to be high class) lived. He and my mother were so happy to look around for houses. As my parents were searching for a home, my oldest brother, Sung Hee, and his wife, my sister-in-law Byeong Sil, visited from Mogpo city, Jeollanam-do. But we soon faced another crisis like a tsunami: on June 25, 1950, the Korean War broke out. No one could believe and accept that that happened in front of us. We all lost. We just did not know what to do; we were incredulous. It was the worst of worsts. We did not know where to look or whom to ask. We were in the deep sea again.

The communists descended upon South Korea quickly. Sung Hee, a police officer in Mogpo, caught the last train before the Han River was closed off, to his home to perform his duties, leaving his wife with us for safety. But Seoul would soon fall to the communists. I could not believe Korea was at war again. We had escaped the communists, believing that everything would be fine in the south, but they were here now, in Seoul, searching for North Korean refugees and Christians. For three days straight, from the mountaintop, my family and I heard gunfire as the communists descended upon Seoul. We never wanted to see the North Korean flag again, but it was hung outside of the Blue House, the residence of the president of South Korea, once the communists conquered the city. We were exhausted, trembling, and scared to death. I was never this scared before, not even compared to when we had crossed the DMZ. I could not figure out how long or how much Sung Kul and I cried in the temple yard until I had no more tears, looking at the North Korean flag waving, the very same flag that we used to see up north. We knew we were going to die. The North Koreans would recognize us as refugees right away because of our dialect. No energy, no strength, no hope was clear; we couldn't escape and felt like we were waiting around to be killed. At that time, I asked if there was a God, how could He let this happen to us? Up until the communists invaded, my brother and I had clung on to hope that things would eventually improve since we were once again united with our family. But seeing the North Korean flag, we could see no sign of God. The impossible became possible, and I lost my faith.

Soon we saw South Korean soldiers escaping from the battlefields near my house on the mountain. They asked us, the civilians, for clothes to pretend that they were not soldiers to escape. Whatever clothing my father and brother had they would give to the fleeing soldiers, while the soldiers left guns and other military equipment behind. My father and Sung Kul hid all the guns under the rocks in the creek at the base of the mountain. (Perhaps the guns might still be there today.) However, one of the soldiers was captured by the North Korean army and paraded around by the ear. They came to our house to search for the gun because the South Korean soldier confessed that he left it near our house. At that time, there was another panic because we knew there were harsh and severe repercussions for all of us. My father had thrown us into a deep dilemma, including this prisoner. The situation at the spot was very urgent, so my father pretended that he did not know what happened to the guns he was hiding. He said that many soldiers and civilians had crossed Inwang Mountain. It was open to everyone, and we could not account for everyone passing through. At this moment, the North Korean armies were standing on the rocks, underneath which all the guns were hidden. Utterly terrified but surprised, I discovered that one of the North Korean soldiers was my former third-grade teacher, who used to be good to me until I left for South Korea. When I recognized him as my teacher, he too was frightened and immediately warned me to not show that we knew each other in front of the other soldiers. It would be death for both of us. But I bravely and impatiently tested him about my dearest friend and my house back in Daegwon-dong. He answered me quietly and softly, saying that my friend went to a labor camp in Ganggye, Pyeonanbuk-do, which was far from my hometown, and my house was changed into a middle school for girls. After telling me this information, he pretended that we were strangers. He firmly and quietly left us, escorting the South Korean soldier away for execution. I watched them walk away, feeling homesick and scared and worried for our life and their lives until they disappeared. This memory is still alive. I can't imagine what became of the South Korean soldier. Who were his mother and father?

From North Korea to America Through Three Wars

The next day, desperate and panicking, my family and I immediately moved from the temple to our church house, far downtown in Hyoja-dong. Shortly after we moved to this house, my sister-in-law, who was only 26 years old, died on July 25, 1950. Realizing that she was not able to go back to her husband in Mogpo due to war, she rapidly became ill, neither eating nor drinking. Emaciated, she was terrified of all the gunfire, cannons, and bombs from the airplanes, too, and started to hallucinate. She soon died in front of me. It was one month after the war had started.

By this time, in Seoul, many people began to evacuate to the countryside for safety. Because there were no working radios or television, I heard through rumors that people were being killed during bombings. My family also moved, to Suwon, an hour by car, but we traveled on foot, and I do not remember how long it took. The all-country roads heading south were filled with people, carrying things on their heads or backs while bombs went off all around. When bombs went off, the people fell flat to the ground and hid under trees. In Seoul, it was hard to buy foods like rice, barley, wheat, etc. Simply, there was no market, and the North Korean army had overrun the city. Everywhere was disaster, with bombings, cannons, death, and hunger. It was so hot outside, and the war was getting worse, with more and more North Korean soldiers arriving. They were quickly changing the social structure of South Korea, turning everything into communism. Maids quit their jobs, not only because there was no more food to serve, but society had changed. They learned that they no longer needed to call the head of the household "madam" but rather "female comrade." Class no longer existed; we were classless or proletarian. Those words reminded me of North Korea. Everyone was suddenly and strictly equal. At that time, one of our neighbors, who was born and raised in South Korea and was used to being called "madam" because she had belonged to the *yangban* class, confessed to my mother that she could finally understand why we had to escape from North Korea. It was little relief for us because the southerners who once looked down on us understood what we had gone through.

Like others, we again had to move to the countryside, far from Suwon to Gyeonggi-do, situated by the Yellow Sea. Fortunately, one of our relatives from a long time ago lived there. This place had no bus

II—The Forgotten War in South Korea

line and could only be reached on foot or by ox to help transport luggage. Of course, there was no electricity either. In this place, we went back to a primitive way of life. For water, the whole village depended on one well, and the roof of the house was constructed with rice straws. At night, everyone used oil lamps. It was completely different than Seoul. During daytime, Sung Kul hid on Gai Sum (개섬), or "Dog Island" in English, which was surrounded by water due to the tide. It was inaccessible without a boat. He spent all day alone, and then at night he rejoined the family. One day, he was so scared because he was late leaving the island, and the tide had already come in. He navigated the sea alone while it was dark without a light to guide him to land. I usually worked for a farm and caught clams, oysters, and fish, depending on the weather and tide. We were all hungry, but catching things very much helped everyone.

In September, we started to hear cannon fire as well as air bombings near Incheon Port. My father and Sung Kul only assumed what was happening in Seoul because we had no telephone, radio, newspaper, or letters. In the middle of September, we heard by rumor that General Douglas MacArthur had arrived in Incheon with the UN Army to liberate Seoul. On September 28, 1950, General MacArthur reclaimed Seoul from the North Koreans. The news, which we'd hoped for, gave us a new life. All agonies, worries, fears, and terrors disappeared with one word: "freedom." This time, "freedom" was different than I used to hear in the past. This was life versus death for all of us. We were excited, with hearts beating faster than ever, jumping, laughing, and shouting. The memories of terror from Inwang Mountain blew away like smoke in the air.

Some people already knew about General MacArthur because he led the defeat of the Japanese in World War II. If this general was involved in the war, the Korean people felt that Korea would have no more war and would be united by him. From this time, many people said that American soldiers were our saviors. My hope simply began to depend on America. I, without any question, wanted to thank America. I do even more than before and deeper. Having hope, we all happily returned to Nusang-dong, the temple on Inwang Mountain, where we continued to live. But soon after, we heard that we had to escape south again because General MacArthur began to withdraw when Chinese troops entered the war and drove the United Nations' forces back to the south. He led the army back to the DMZ, which has been the dividing line between the north and south since. Now Jangdan and Gaeseong are officially part of North Korea.

    We again had no hope for our future and had to depend on my father. Many people tried to go to Busan or Deagu in the south to survive under the South Korean soldiers, but my father felt that we should go to Mogpo, Jeollanam-do, where my oldest brother was a police officer. He thought that during the war, the whole family should get together. Every road south was filled with people of all ages on foot carrying things on their heads and backs, as much as they could, crying, complaining, and being helpless in the cold. Whenever people reached a village or town, they went into the houses, eating whatever they could find or what was left behind by previous owners who had already fled south. On our own journey, we stopped in an abandoned home and found jars full of kimchi buried underground. Starving, we unearthed the jars and ate the kimchi, and it was the best kimchi I'd ever eaten. I've never been able to make kimchi that was as delicious as the one we found at the empty home. Like everyone else who was fleeing, we ate quickly, rested, and then continued to the last destination, like where we were in the tent in Jangdan in 1948. But my father picked up my older sister Sung Sook with her two-year-old son on the way south, headed to Mogpo where the road was called Honam Line. It was January 4, 1951, which has become known as the January 4 Retreat, and all citizens were alerted to retreat south in the cold, ahead of the Third Battle of Seoul. My family was in Joenju, Jeonllabuk-do, where there was a big tunnel that no one could walk through because it was so long and dark. My family and I got on the top of the train, which was the last train from Joenju to Sunchon, exposed to the cold without any seat belts or safety precautions, but for some reason, my father could not join us. When the train started to move, Sung Sook fell from the top to the ground. She quickly climbed back on top of the train with us, and we arrived at Suncheon train station in Jeollanam-do. On the way, we passed through Jiri Mountain tunnel: long and dark, our faces dirty from the smoke of the train billowing.

    Without my father, we all arrived at Suncheon train station. Everyone clambered off the train, and we did not know what to do in this situation. Our family was separated from my father without any way of knowing how to find him, and we had no place to go for the night to sleep. Our fate was like chaff in the air. It was freezing outside, and there was no refugee camp either. We knocked on the doors of all the houses, asking for a place to stay but were turned away. It was not only us, but everyone else who arrived on this train. Fortunately, a pregnant woman welcomed my family and me to stay in her home even though we didn't know her at all.

Our hostess delivered a boy while we were staying in her house. My sister and mother assisted with the delivery. One morning, my mother looked out through the window and saw a man who was begging for food. Then she sensed that the man could be my father. She asked me to go to him and call out "father" to confirm it was him. He was my father! Immediately, after hearing my voice, he hugged me and cried hard. I couldn't stop crying. He explained how he got lost trying to join us on top of the train in Jeonju. He had to go back inside the station to ask a question, not knowing how soon the train would leave. But the train had already started to move, and an officer stopped him from getting on the train, even though the officer knew that we, his family, were on it. He then left alone, hungry, but his will was only to find the family. He wrapped straw rope around his waist, from his chest to hip, for strength. He prayed to God for his safety, reciting Psalm 23, and he decided to go through the mountain tunnel we had passed through to get to Suncheon. He was told by people that the tunnel was occupied by the communist partisans and tigers because it was long, and nobody had used the route for a long time. But my father was determined to find his family. Starving, with no light or directions, he trekked through the tunnel. Then he bent and crawled like a baby because he could not stand or walk with no light inside of the tunnel. While he was counting the beams, he was able to concentrate on moving forward. He said that the more he moved forward, the stillness was deeper, and it was scary to be alone. It was really a deep darkness was what he said. He could not remember how long it took, but he felt that the light was coming soon. He felt that he could live. Then he sensed that his undergarments were all wet, but he was so thankful that he was not trapped by any partisan group or tigers. He sincerely prayed to God on his knees after he made it out of the tunnel alive. On the other side, he began to beg for food while following the rail because he figured that we might be in some area of Suncheon by the train station. That's when my mother saw him on the streets. We were all happy to find my father with no phone, letters, or talking, hungry and cold, exposed to the elements as a beggar.

From there, my father found a way for us to travel the train rails from Suncheon to Mogpo with a manual handcar that was roughly the size of a van. Finally, we arrived in Mogpo and found a refugee camp. The camp was much better than the Buddhist temple in Seoul because it was run by American missionaries, and fortunately, we didn't face discrimination in Mogpo because we were among many residents from Seoul, fellow southerners. Soon after, Sung Sook got sick, suffering difficulty breathing with pain inside of her chest and edema on her face, abdomen, and legs, all because of her fall from the train in Jeonju, and died at 25 years old. It was an internal injury, and she had no access to medical treatment from a doctor or hospital. She left behind her two-year-old son and never got to see her husband, Dong Hwa, again because he had been conscripted into the South Korean National Guard. He did not know that his wife was dead. They were so close and loved each other fiercely. My sister had crossed the DMZ about two years earlier, escaping war and death, but died from an accident while fleeing as a refugee. My mother could not take it, and she asked, "Why do you have to die in this way?" My mother kept crying and lost her eyesight after my sister died. Then, two months after Sung Sook's death, my father died suddenly at the refugee camp in April 1951, after eating something outside that made him fatally ill.

We all felt hopeless when my father died because he was our family's breadwinner and leader. With his and Sung Sook's deaths, we lost everything that mattered, our family, and did not know what to do. Although so many families had lost their loved ones, we essentially lost two at once and felt more helpless. We just cried, cried, and cried until we had no more tears or strength left. It still brings tears to my eyes remembering Sung Sook's death, leaving her son and missing her husband during the war. My oldest brother, the police officer, could not care for us because he became so depressed after he learned his wife had died, that he could not see her again. Another brother, Sung Kul, was enlisted in the marines in South Korea before January 4, 1951.

II—The Forgotten War in South Korea

I wondered how we would ever continue living. I had watched my sister die and my father, too; it was the second time I saw dead bodies of my family members. They were colorless, unresponsive, and cold to the touch. How could such a strong man die? I wondered why I was still alive. It was too much for me to handle as a child. I was numb. My mother was likewise devastated and blamed herself for their deaths. I recall her crying out, "What did I do wrong?" Even worse, not only had she lost her husband, but since she was now a widow, society would look down on her. She had no formal education, no source of income. She had been completely dependent on my father. We needed rations for food, relying on the government for help, and would have to figure out how to make a living going forward.

Before my father died, he enrolled me in fifth grade at Subu Elementary School in the camp. I continued to attend the school after his passing. After fifth grade, my mother, younger brother, and I moved to the place where we used to stay with my father during the war in September 1950. In this area, I finished sixth grade, while my mother began to work as a farmhand. After I finished sixth grade, I began to work alongside my mother, and we were paid in barley. For one day's work, my mother received one doe (되) of barley, equal to 1.6 kg, whereas I received half the amount since I was only a teenager. One hot day while I was working diligently in the fields, one of my former classmates from sixth grade who now went to Sookmyoung Girl's High School in Seoul visited me in her white shirt and blue skirt uniform. She was on her way home to visit her mother during summer vacation and wanted to see me. She said that she'd been thinking of me during the schoolyear. We wept together because I couldn't go to school with her, and I was so envious of her uniform. She looked so high class and had the life that I missed and wanted. At that time, I began to feel that I was so different than she was, because I did not wear the same uniform. Instead, it was like holding a short-handled hoe with dirty hands in the cornfields. There was a visible and direct class difference even at that young age. That made me sad, but I had to keep weeding.

When winter came, we had no jobs. Finally, my mother became a housemaid, and I did, too, moving into the different houses. Then I had to work in a home factory, making fried tofu for sushi and rice cakes as a maid. It was tough to get up early every morning in winter, preparing the fire to warm water and the house. At this time, I was about seventeen years old, not attending any school. Sung Kul, who was a marine veteran, wearing the uniform of a marine corps officer, came to pick me up for school one day while I was working in the kitchen. He introduced himself to the owner of the house, a woman, and explained to her why he'd come. When Sung Kul saw me at that factory, with bleeding, cracked hands in cold ice water, we both burst into tears as he held my hands. It was the first time we'd seen one another since Mogpo. He and I left for Jinhae, Gyeongsangnam-do, where Sung Kul camped, and he prepared for my enrollment in ninth grade at Jinhae Girls' Middle School. The school's policy did not allow older students to be in the same class as the younger girls, so when the school asked Sung Kul for my age upon enrollment, he claimed that I'd attended another school in Seoul for seventh and eighth grades. He fabricated my age and transcripts, saying this was an exceptional case due to the war. So I had to be in the ninth grade without learning the English alphabet. In English class on my first day at school, I was called on by the teacher to read the English textbook aloud, but I couldn't do it. I kept quiet and sat down, crying. When I came home, I told Sung Kul that I did not want to go back to school again the next day. He and I sobbed hard for a long time. It was pitiful but touching. Finally, he put his hands on my head and prayed that I would find the strength to continue going to school or that someone would help me. He taught me the alphabet and how to use the English dictionary to learn vocabulary. I often slept only three to four hours each night throughout all those years, and it paid off. I succeeded and was able to attend Duk Sung Girls' High School back in Seoul, now liberated, the following year.

Still, our family situation was desperate. Sung Kul was transferred from Jinhae city to near the DMZ, and my mother had to keep going to another city to work as a maid, while my younger brother, Sung Duk, stayed in Jinhae with a friend to continue middle school. My family was separated, and we had no way to stay in touch because no one had a permanent address. I would continue to survive without my family because I had to go to Seoul to continue high school. I don't know how I persisted without my mother and brother. And once again, I had no place to stay. But thankfully, one of our relatives offered for me to stay with them for a short time because they knew our desperate situation very well, although they did not have any extra space for me. It was awfully kind, but it was very uncomfortable to stay there, especially when it came to eating and sleeping because I essentially became one of their children. Thankfully, soon one of Sung Kul's friends introduced me as a private tutor to one family who had three daughters ranging first to eighth grades and they were looking for a live-in tutor. The eighth-grader, Sook, had been having a problem with enuresis (bed-wetting at night) for a long time. Also, her schoolwork as not great. The parents of Sook had been concerned about her for a long time and had gone through many other private tutors who had been university students.

Usually, to be a private tutor you need to be a university student. Unfortunately, the tutors, who shared a room with Sook, did not stay long enough, nor did they get along well with Sook because of the nightly smell of the urine. Now, the parents were fully aware of the problems with the university students from their past experiences. With these problems, they had a different approach to hire a tutor for Sook at this time. For a trial, they preferred a high school student like me. I was a perfect fit for this situation, which was rare as a high school student. I felt I was so fortunate. It appeared all my frustration disappeared. Finally, I was able to go to school, not worrying about eating and sleeping every day.

Being Sook's private tutor for a short time, I was so surprised with Sook's English grade, which I couldn't understand at all. Sook's English grade went up quickly. I had never been a teacher in English, but it looked like I had become a good teacher. In fact, I had struggled with learning English in the past, but things happened. I was not sure what I had done for Sook. One day, her school's principal visited us to find how Sook suddenly improved her grade in English. The principal thought that Sook was cheating in some way. Sook's mother thought Sook would be in big trouble with the school, but the principal was impressed by how much I'd helped her improve. She said that I must be a good teacher. From this comment, Sook's parents treated me like a queen, which I was uncomfortable with because I had never been in this situation. I was used to being looked down on.

But it did not last long. Although we still slept in the same room, Sook did not study with me anymore. In fact, her feelings toward me changed drastically. Her enuresis worsened. When she woke up wet in the early morning, she was rude and mean to me. Sook became more disrespectful and uncooperative. A previous maid told me that Sook was now behaving as she had with the previous tutors, which led to the tutors leaving. But I had no other choice, nor could I resist. Rather, I began to worry about her grade in English and behaviors because her grade was declining. Gradually, Sook did not pay attention to me like she used to. She became sensitive and impatient, refusing to listen to me anymore. She indirectly looked down on me as a high school student, wearing the same clothes every day, whereas she had worn a more prestigious uniform at the private school she attended. One day, I had to borrow her mother's jacket to attend to my school affair, but Sook told her mother to no longer let me borrow her clothes. Sook's parents soon started to treat me differently as well. After they realized how poor my family was, their attitude and behavior toward me were different, and one day I overheard Sook's mother mocking me for being poor to her friends. It stung. The family no longer treated me as a teacher but rather as a maid. I began to sense that I was in the wrong place, but I couldn't leave because our family members were all spread out. I had no place to go. At this point, I began to feel like I was a housemaid again who had to accept the situation.

My struggles accumulated like mountains, and frustrations filled inside of me. I had no other choice except to sleep and eat with the endless smell of urine. Living like this, I could not have any hope, nor could I dream like other high school girls. My only dream at that time was to get out of the house and to be united with my mother and younger brother and to eat in our own home, no matter how it looked, bad or small. Since I had finished sixth grade, I had been away from my family, not eating together. I missed home so much. It was a dream. I just wanted to finish high school and find a job to live with my family. I never wanted to be or feel like a maid ever again. I was dragging myself to the end of the senior year, only hoping that Sook would perform better, but it looked impossible.

While I was frustrated with Sook and her family, one day my brother Sung Kul suggested that I enroll in nursing school after graduating from high school. The minute I heard the word "nursing," I was frightened. Without thinking, I simply said, "No." I just wanted to finish high school and find a job, maybe as a typist or a kind of clerk but not a nurse. This word, nursing, made me feel like I'd be a maid my whole life. I said to myself that I would try not to be a maid forever after high school. I felt that I already had disgraceful feelings being a housemaid in the past. It was an unavoidable situation during the war, but now that the war was over, I refused to take low-class work again. It was sad and shameful for me and my family. I thought I could do or be more than a nurse. Then, I urgently wanted to be home with my mother like other families.

When I heard the word "nurse" from my brother, of course I did not talk about my feelings and struggles at all. It was no use to tell him because he knew well what and how much I had been in difficult situations for a long time, ever since crossing the DMZ and my father's death. Understanding our family situation, Sung Kul had taken on the role of our father for all of us, which was untraditional. My oldest brother, Sung Hee, should've taken on the role, but he was unable to do it. Sung Kul knew well how our lives had been completely turned upside down once we left home. Since then, we only had sufferings and ongoing miseries, and he worried about my future and wished me better than the past. Our family situation was at the bottom based on the Confucian social structure. I did not want, nor could I accept the situation, but I had obeyed too well, all the way through until now. Sung Kul was hurt by my grievous hardships and sad because he could do nothing for me at that time. He worried about me more than himself. He was a veteran because he got injured during the Korean War, on the battlefield in the winter of 1951. In his worrying about my future, he searched for what I should do as a profession. Just in time, he had a friend who had been in the United States and collected information on nursing from him, which was a respected profession unlike in South Korea. At that time, whoever went to America was well respected and admired by the people in South Korea because America was known as a paradise on the planet, and it was not easy to go to. But I did not take his suggestion, nor did I try to understand it either because I believed that nurses were nothing more than doctors' helpers. That concept strongly came to me and hit me before I took Sung Kul's suggestion. Without taking time to understand what it meant to be a nurse, I simply resented nursing, considering nurses to be a helper, maid, servant, etc. Also, going to America seemed impossible for me because my English was not at all strong. I immediately and strongly refused his idea. My dream was so simple: to live with my mother as well as my younger brother, Sung Duk. Missing and wishing for home for a long time, I did not even want to go to college. But then, I knew well why Sung Kul suggested that I go to nursing school. I was in a dilemma: to go or not to go to nursing school. I asked friends what I should do, but most people naturally thought like me that nursing school was a kind of maid in the doctor's office or hospital, per Confucian cultural views. People were asking me why I considered studying nursing as a university student; they actually asked, "Is there even a nursing course in university?" I was not able to answer them easily either. In addition, I did not want to live as a maid, with its low status, for my entire life.

Sung Kul strongly advised me again to go to nursing school for my future. It offered the opportunity to go to the United States as a professional at a time when people couldn't move there. Usually, the smart students had to take examinations to go to America and were treated so highly by the public and at jobs as well. In addition, I knew that America was our family's savior from the Korean War. Of course, I wanted to go there badly, but I knew that I was not qualified to go there right away. America was a dream place for everyone. In addition, Sung Kul truly cared for me and didn't want me to turn out as just a doctor's helper. As I considered my brother's concern for me, I was able to understand and grew more inclined toward accepting his suggestion. Finally, I said to him weakly, "Yes." He brightened and said to me that time was running out for applying to nursing schools, and only Ewha Womans University for nursing was still open. He rushed to get the papers for me and coerced me to take the enrollment examination in 1959.

III

The Reluctant Nursing Student

I took the enrollment exam for Ewha Womans University Nursing Department, hoping that I would fail, but I passed. There was now no way that I could avoid going to nursing school to obtain my baccalaureate of science in nursing (BSN). Although the BSN was very important in the nursing world, I didn't care because I had no interest in nursing.

Rather than celebrating this milestone, I had sunk deeper into the sea of anxiety because I would need to pay tuition somehow, and I would also have to study for a career that I didn't want. Additionally, I couldn't afford fashionable clothes like the other university students. Ewha Womans University students were particularly well known for being fashionable, wearing tailored clothing from Sears in the United States. Back then, women who purchased clothes from Sears were proud and often bragged about their wardrobe. For me, buying such clothes was impossible. Since the only pair of shoes that I owned were sneakers that were part of my high school uniform, a friend of mine gave me a nicer pair of shoes that used to belong to her sister. However, they did not fit my feet and instead chafed and tore up my heels. I had to walk barefoot, holding these fancier shoes at my side to go to class. Not only that, I carried a worn-out book bag, which was also given to me by my friend. I was embarrassed to be in this situation. Escaping poverty felt like an insurmountable feat, with only further tough times lurking on the horizon. My agonies continued to mount, reaching up into the sky, because I would have to continue to stay with Sook. Ewha Womans University mandated that students move into the dormitory from junior year, which was two years away. Without another place to live, I would need to share a room with Sook for two more years. She was highly fashionable and already looked down on me; she would be even crueler to me once I announced that I would be attending nursing school. It was close to hell, but I was stuck with no other choice.

Even if I finished my degree in nursing, there was no guarantee that I would go to the United States. Sung Kul claimed that if I went to the States, I would find success as a nurse, unlike at home in Korea, where nursing was viewed as a lesser profession. My dream felt like a wispy cloud dissipating in the sky. It was a fate that I could neither understand nor accept. I was simply helpless and hopeless, and I became depressed. My mind urged me to reject becoming a nurse. The more I contemplated my past and future, I knew it was not right for me. All I wanted was to eat my mother's kimchi with my family—although everyone made kimchi, no one's kimchi tasted like my mother's. I yearned to be in my own home again, just for one day, but that was a pipe dream. Then what was my reason to be alive? Why didn't I die during the Korean War? Who could I blame for my current situation? The more I thought, the more I found unanswered because it was impossible to know the causes. I believed it was fate not to be dead during the war or crossing the DMZ. It was inconceivable to find out reasons. Once I felt that I was lucky and thankful to be alive through all the difficulties, but now I felt guilty about being alive. I had to accept as it was with questioning, asking, or complaining. But my resistance was running out, and my patience was nearly gone. I began to review the past about what and how I had lived. The reviewing was simple: to be born in North Korea and then to live through the Korean War. In my memories, I couldn't remember what our family or myself did wrong. Rather, I asked myself, should we have stayed in North Korea and not looked for democracy? Obviously, I did not know what democracy meant at that time. I just copied the word "democracy" by the people's language. Once, I'd had a family and a home back in the north but had lost it all in pursuit of freedom. Now, I had no past, home, family, or dreams. Is this the price of freedom? There was no one to listen to my complaints or answer my questions; additionally, there was no one to console me, support me anyway. No one asked why Korea was divided in two, nor did anyone think to ask if I was suffering. Practically everyone just accepted the result of war

III—The Reluctant Nursing Student

without question; was I the only one asking about it? My mind and thoughts were filled with unanswered questions, and I continued to blame myself. I felt that I was born for this suffering, to keep questioning these things.

Even now, this feeling brings tears into my eyes. Talking to Sung Kul, who is now 90 and living in Chicago, I know that he feels the same way. All these terrible things were going on around us and still occur today. I couldn't control anything. I was just Sung Chon from Daegwon-dong. I still had no idea how I ended up in this situation since I left North Korea, and my former childhood felt like a life that someone else had lived.

My feelings plummeted deeper into the abyss, and I could no longer persist through these grievous hardships. I no longer had the energy to endure pain. I lost myself; I had no values or any desire to live. I only thought about giving up everything and committing suicide. I only considered how to die. From that point, I felt like I had no outside, inside, past, present, or future. I wondered, after I died, what would happen to my body? Should I die by the river? On a mountain? While I considered ways to die, I suddenly thought about how my mother would deal with my death. I clearly remembered when my sister Sung Sook died during the Korean War in 1951, my mother had lost her eyesight, and she was so heart broken. How could I ever give my mother another blow? With this question, I was alerted to my mother's inevitable sorrow. She was a pure, loving mother and adjusted to all given situations, complaining of Kim Il-sung only. She loved me more than I could ever love her, and my love for her was endless. That love dragged me away from suicide to live in this world longer and stronger. The power of love stoked my blood to run faster to fill my heart.

With a changed mind, I informed Sook and her parents that I had decided to go to Ewha Womans University for nursing. They were so glad that I made it into that school, but as I assumed, they asked me why I chose to study nursing. They were even surprised that there was a nursing course offered by the university. I explained that I had heard about all the possibilities in the nursing world, which changed their attitudes toward me. Whereas they initially looked down on me because I was poor, the lowest social status according to Confucius, they now treated me with more respect because I was going to attend such a prestigious university. In fact, her parents asked me to stay longer because they saw Sook was changing for the worse and could not find another tutor who could tolerate her. But Sook was different from her parents because she expected me to act like other university students, following fashions and other trends, not studying nursing. She'd become a snob and continued to look down on me with her stereotyped attitude toward poor people and studying nursing rather than medicine. But I changed my attitude toward her rudeness, acting kinder and more accepting, even though Sook refused to change. When she spoke down to me, I remember thinking, one day I will be different than who I am now. Finally, the time came for me to move into the dormitory, which was located near the hospital. After four years, I gladly left Sook, who had grown taller than me since starting high school. She was preparing for college, and now aware of how helpful I'd been, she desperately wanted me to still be her tutor—her bed-wetting problem remained, too—but it was time for me to go. In the end, her parents shared their appreciation. Their praise lifted me up, making my patience and efforts worth it.

Staying in the dormitory was quite a different experience. As nursing students, we ate together and slept together, eight nursing students stuffed into a room with only one light on the ceiling. Our sleeping beds were bunk beds, but I at least had my own bed, which made me feel good. For me, no longer stuck with Sook, it was liberation, and I was finally comfortable. But I had another complicated problem because I was older than my cohort. Traditionally, classes consisted of students of the same age, but I was three to four years older than my peers. It was the first time I was thrown into such a situation. According to the traditional Korean language system, age difference is very important; how to recognize a person, who he or she is, and how to address them is related to age as well as educational background, social status, and family background. The Korean language is crucial to one's identity. In addition, the Korean way of counting age isn't like the American way. If you were born on December 31, the next day, January 1, you will be counted as two years old. One year makes quite a difference between two people. Koreans must speak respectfully to someone who is one year older. Usually, my classmates did not need to pay any attention to age because they were all essentially the same

III—The Reluctant Nursing Student

age. I was much older and could be their older sister. Therefore, they felt very uncomfortable talking to or having any conversation with me because they felt confused speaking to me in a respectful way because I was their peer, at their same level in class. So I had problems communicating with my classmates. I felt alone and very uneasy whenever I was in class with some kind of inferiority and shame. Not only that, but based on the culture, they asked questions like "Where are you from?" or "Where were you born?"

None of these questions made it easy to get along with my classmates. Naturally, I was separated from them and was frustrated when learning and building relationships with my peers. I couldn't keep my self-esteem like other students who wanted to learn more about nursing. My background and current situation together made me less interested in studying nursing. I once again had to navigate these cultural concepts alone. I dislike Confucianism and its impact on the Korean language because English is more casual. Regardless of class, social status, or age, everyone, from a newborn and to an elder, is simply referred to as "you." At that time, I did not understand how the meaning of words like "you" and "I" differed in the English and Korean languages. Later, I felt that English words were more egalitarian, indicating a degree of equality between two persons, regardless of age or social rank. For example, in English, between a one-year-old child and an 80-year-old man, they were able to communicate using the same word, just "you" and "me" or "I." This indicated clearly, they are at the same level as a person not counting age. This meaning led me to learn English more for my own good. In addition, this concept could be related to the democratic idea indicating that everybody is equal, regardless of age, gender, or social status. When I sensed this significance, I was fascinated with elation for learning English. In addition, I was enlightened by the meaning of the words, that it contained and represented in many ways such as the social classes, equality, and the level of intelligence of humans. Recognizing this enlightenment, I respected my father who was so strict and firm to emphasize the need to learn the language properly.

But with support from Sung Kul, I was able to continue to study despite this language issue and my lack of interest in nursing. Throughout my time at Ewha Womans University, I learned to be independent and resilient. I even received a scholarship from the school due to my diligence. In 1963, I finally graduated and earned my BSN. After graduation, I obtained my registered nurse license in Korea. Formally, I was ready to work as a nurse.

By this time, I had met my future husband, Insok Yoo, through mutual acquaintances. He was an office worker at a construction company, who was supporting his family and his widowed mother, Young Kyu. As a young man, he was gentle looking but had a strong figure, with a deep mind, and was very thoughtful. He was from an impoverished background with a younger sister and brother who needed support from him. When I met him, I felt very comfortable, which was quite different than I'd been in my past. Until then, my life was pulled and dragged into a new situation without me having a say. Then I had to adjust and act like I did not have any complaints or wishes. I'd had no dreams or hopes of how to live in the future, but meeting Insok perked me up, and I was refreshed to have a new life. We were able to communicate about poverty from the war and understand the current situations without feeling shame or the need to explain ourselves. He did not show any uneasiness like the traditional way of thinking, which was very uncommon at that time, but I felt he was quite open minded and had a positive way of thinking, both of which I needed desperately for support. So I felt that I could share with him in my future happily. I loved

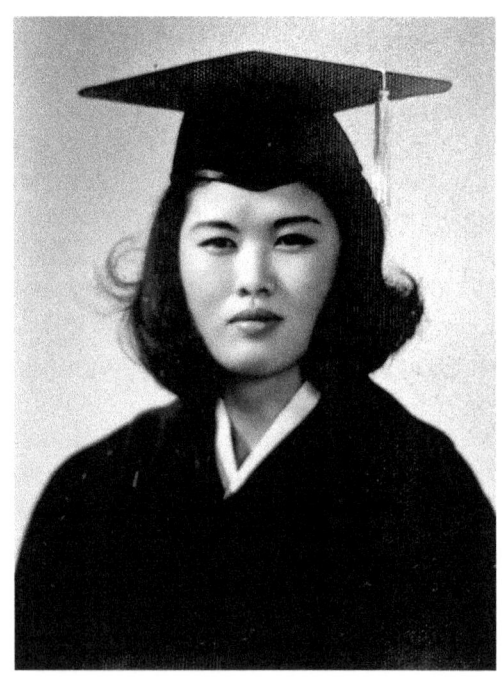

Sung Yoo's graduation from the nursing program at the very highly regarded Ewha Womans University, Seoul, South Korea, 1963.

him more for coming from such a poor condition because I had been in that condition, too. But everyone thought it would be much better for me to marry a rich man. Additionally, Insok was not a Christian, whereas my family were still fiercely devout despite all we'd been through. Then, I no longer believed in God, Jesus, and the Holy Spirit. Religion played no part in my life—I simply believed in myself—and Insok didn't really care about religion, which made me comfortable. Another issue was that I was already older than I should be for an unmarried woman at that time, according to Korean trends. Insok did not mind my age, a major benefit for me because I was not thinking about marriage either because our family situation made it impossible to pay for a wedding, even though I would've liked to get married. It was far away for me.

Sung Kul had a plan for me after nursing school. He searched for a man who was looking for a wife. Sung Kul wished that I would be in much better financial condition because he knew what I had been through since crossing the DMZ when I was ten years old. He told me that I should no longer suffer financial hardship and everything else. He told me that he loved me more than himself. So when he heard about Insok, who was so different than his wishes, he strongly rejected Insok, ordering me to stop seeing him. Yes, of course, I understood Sung Kul's view, but until now, my way of my life, I was not happy at all. If I married someone who I did not like or love only for money, then it would have been worse than my past. That was my understanding and belief at that time. I hoped only one thing, which was marriage should be what I want to do. Then, for some reason, I did not mind that Insok's family was indigent. Rather, I felt that I would have more energy for doing everything. At that time, I did not read the Bible, but this quote captures how I felt: "There is nothing love cannot face; there is no limit to its faith, its hope, its endurance" (1 Corinthians 13:7).

Having these feelings, I strongly persisted in continuing the relationship with Insok, who told me, "If we are together, we will create a new life, from poverty to prosperity." I felt that these words were more than money and my driving force. I already felt that I gained the deep meaning of power from these words. I had never expected to have this plentiful relief and comfort by his words. I was ready to do anything with him and felt very content in my heart. I even did not want to talk about the man who was arranged by Sung Kul, a banker with a nice house. That made me nervous. I sensed that if I married this man, I would have to obey him for the rest of my life as a maid. I began to have a big clash with Sung Kul.

IV

The Vietnam War

In the 1960s, South Korea suffered an outbreak of tuberculosis (TB), the worst in all of Asia.

The World Health Organization (WHO) spearhead a special project to control the TB epidemic. One of the studies oversaw giving the Bacillus Calmette-Guérin (BCG) vaccine to children and adults who were shown to be at lower risk of TB for prevention of the probability after undergoing chest X-rays. The BCG vaccine study had two teams: an urban team in Seoul and a rural team in Bucheon, Gyeonggi-do. In the spring of 1964, I was hired to work as a nurse—called a BCG nurse—in Bucheon, an hour by train from my home.

That was my first job as a nurse, and I chose this position as a public health nurse because it did not require me to give bedside care to patients or wear a hospital nurse's white uniform. I did not need to work nights, weekends, or holidays. I looked like a normal working person in an office, which made me feel better about my decision to become a nurse. Wearing the all-white nurse's uniform was not what I had wanted. If I had worked at the hospital instead, I would have had to work the nightshift, in uniform, which I did not like. While previously working the nightshift as a nursing student, I envied the patients who slept in their beds, while I was forced to stay awake. Physically, it was hard to work at night as well as during the weekends. I never considered the care, what it meant, and what nursing was all about. I did not think of asking, nor was I interested in knowing, those things at that time. I was still reluctant to be a nurse and just followed the requirements of the curricula and clinical practice to get a paycheck. Truth be told, I was narrow-minded and ignorant, being unhappy about my chosen profession.

From North Korea to America Through Three Wars

But Sung Kul was beyond happy that I had become a working woman. For the first time since the war ended, we all gathered as a family in Sangdo-dong, outside of Seoul, in a house built by Sung Kul and Sung Duk. They built the house with bricks made by Sung Kul, who'd learned the technique while in the army. They, themselves, made all the bricks from clay in the local area. The house lacked wood beams and steel for support, so when it rained, we worried that the house would sink into the ground. But my mother told us, "I don't care how it looks or that it's not done well because I am able to freely stretch out my legs and arms at night as much as I want and can be comfortable, without worrying about anyone else's feelings." She had shared a bed for so many years with discomfort. It was such a long journey to finally be in our own home once again. I recalled the song "Home, Sweet Home" by Sir Henry Rowley Bishop which explained well my feelings. Also, that feeling reminded me of when I heard it the first time in Pyongyang in North Korea. We all surely felt that we were joyous in our sweet home.

We simply loved living in our home. The experience of loving our home taught me about what a sweet home was. The teaching was that we owned the house, not caring about it looked and how it was built but only that it was our own. That feeling made us comfortable; there was no more fear but relaxation. Even as we ate my mother's cooking together at one table for the first time in forever, we couldn't escape feelings of sadness because my father had always been the head of our family, but he was no longer with us. My mother's cooking revived the past, and the food, though what we were used to and had grown up eating, felt new to us, and we embraced our traditional way of dining, talking, and sleeping again. It had been such a long journey for this moment of normalcy.

The following year, I married Insok despite strong objections from Sung Kul. He completely felt that he lost all his love, wishes, and endurance for me. He had been working harder than my father or any other brothers to give us a better life, and he desperately hoped for a better living condition for me in the future. He knew how hard it might be for me to marry into an impoverished family with a widowed mother-in-law, Young Kyu, who'd become a widow at 29 years old, in 1948, with four children, because her husband died suddenly

IV—The Vietnam War

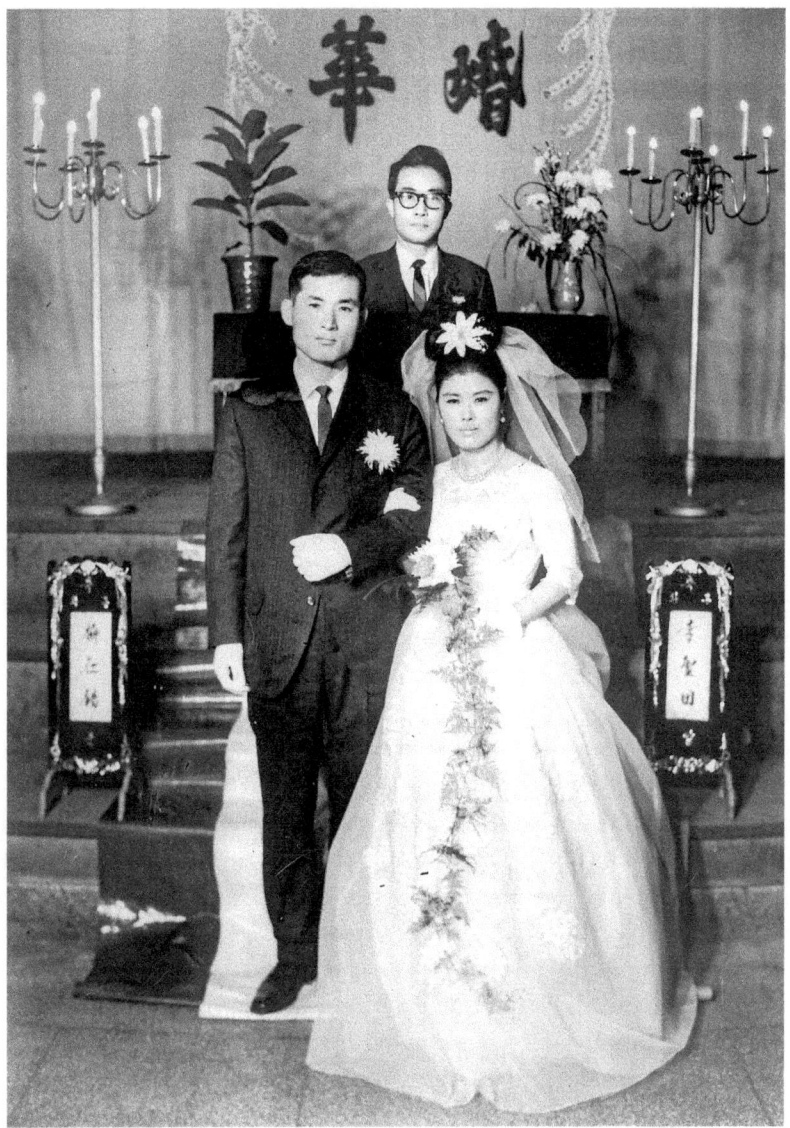

Wedding of Sung Yoo and Insok Yoo, December 6, 1964.

due to a stomach ulcer, an ailment that was unable to be remedied at that time. Since Insok had been ten years old, his mother had been the sole breadwinner. Sung Kul could not accept my decision to marry against his wishes after all his efforts. He decided not to attend my wedding. Equally, Young Kyu had cried because she hoped to have a daughter-in-law from a wealthy family, not me, whose birthplace was North Korea. Traditionally, northern women were seen as having poorer manners than southern women. She cared deeply about these customs and had in her mind the perfect image of who should be her daughter-in-law. I was also born in the Year of the Tiger, whereas Insok was born in the Year of the Ox, according to the Chinese zodiac. Tigers were seen as stronger than oxen, and it was feared that as an ox, Insok would die young. Moreover, females were not supposed to be stronger than males. Chinese culture, specifically Confucianism and zodiac, was truly ingrained into Korean culture, although I was not traditional, which was very rare at the time. But elders were fierce traditionalists. As a widow, Young Kyu understandably was even more reluctant about the wedding than my brother.

Although neither my brother nor Insok's mother supported our marriage, my mother was on our side because Insok had made a good impression. He was like my late-sister's husband who was so good to her; their resemblance was almost uncanny. My mother regretted the political situation that forced us to flee to South Korea because she could offer no dowry. She came to the wedding empty handed. She was so sad at that point, but she was happy for my wedding. Together, we cried because she couldn't provide me with anything. Although I fully understood why, she again blamed Kim Il-sung (she always called him "nom, gae-sae-kki," or what essentially means "horrible man, worthless child," one of the worst insults in Korean), as habit, for us losing everything in North Korea. On December 6, 1964, Insok and I married in the most economical way. At the last minute, Sung Kul ended up attending the nuptials. On that day, he was supposed to escort President Park Chung-hee to the airport for his historical flight to visit South Korean miners and nurses working in West Germany. The president was set to depart at noon, while my wedding was at 3:00 p.m. Sung Kul showed up for the wedding after all and even walked me down the aisle, with both of us in tears. Unfortunately, my makeup was a mess, but I did not care. Despite these circumstances and all the hardships so far, I did not mind at all because I was sincerely happy. Many years later, after we moved to the United States as Sung Kul suggested when I applied to Ewha Womans University to become a nurse,

IV—The Vietnam War

Insok and I visited Sung Kul to celebrate his 90th birthday. We reminisced about my wedding day, now laughing and thankful that God helped us carry on all these years. Sung Kul confessed about his feelings on our wedding day. He said, "I followed the chicken hard, but the chicken just flew away. I felt totally empty in my heart."

One year after we married, Insok and I welcomed a beautiful daughter, naming her Hyen Ju. The birth of my first child brought us closer, and we all lived in harmony. My mother-in-law was the happiest person ever when she saw her granddaughter, her first grandchild. Since she'd been a widow, Hyen Ju's birth revitalized her. Everyone noticed the change in her demeanor, and we would comment, "Nobody loves their granddaughter as much as Young Kyu." In the meantime, I was transferred from Bucheon, Gyeonggi-do to the National Institutes of Health (NIH) in Seoul and joined the teaching staff in the service program of school nurses run by the WHO in 1965. It all looked good on the surface of our lives, working days in the office as part of the teaching staff in Seoul, but inside it wasn't. Our financial situation became worse with fixed incomes, increased expenses with the new baby, and accrued debts from wedding costs despite us pursuing the cheapest option. Although I tolerated our thrifty way of life, there seemed to be no way out. Then, coincidently, the Vietnam War heated up and the South Korean government was seeking administrators, technicians, and laborers, such as construction workers, to send to Vietnam, offering generous compensation. My husband thought, "This is the chance to pay off all our debts." He applied as an administrator for the high salary since it was no comparison to what his company offered. But the risk of injury or death was high. It was less than two years after we married and presented a huge dilemma—to go or not to go—but he bravely went to Vietnam to pay off our debts because there were no other options.

While Insok was in Vietnam, my mother passed away due to high blood pressure problems, having a stroke three days and then again six months after my daughter was born. At the time of her death, my mother was living in the brick house that my brothers had built outside of Seoul, while I was living with Young Kyu, not too far from the blue presidential house. My mother always helped our neighbors in North Korea as well as in South Korea despite being poor. She defied

From North Korea to America Through Three Wars

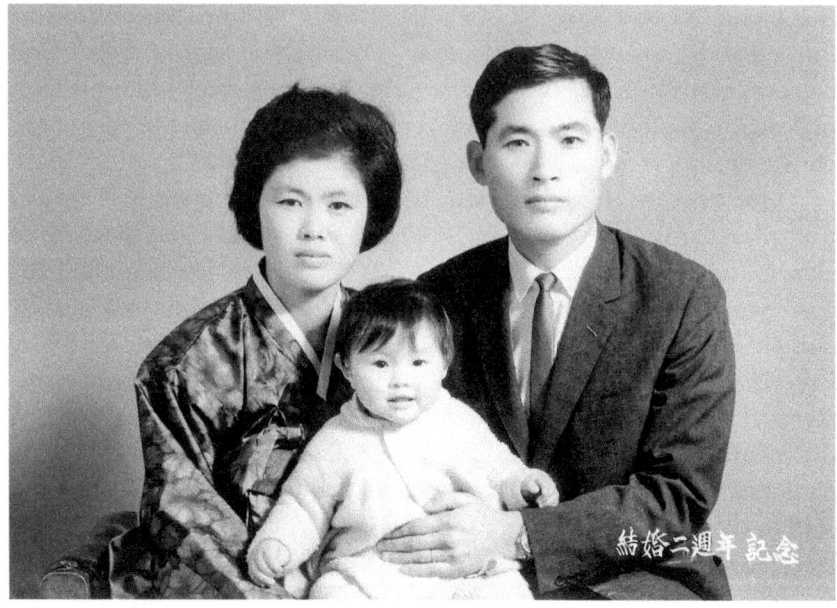

Family portrait before going to Vietnam, August 1968. Their daughter, Hyen Ju, stayed in Korea with Sung Yoo's mother-in-law.

social class ideals and would share food with beggars. As her body lay in the brick house after she passed, one beggar whom she fed stopped by to pay her condolences and mourn with us. She lamented my mother's death, wondering why my mother was taken before her. My mother used to share the cold or warm foods with her in one place together, which was not common based on the cultural concept related to social class between beggar and host. My mother was buried at the church cemetery where we North Koreans sought to find our loved ones who had also fled the communists. As I got older, I missed my mother more and more, recognizing that she truly loved her neighbors as the Bible preached. She had pure love for our family until she died.

The following year, the Korean government announced the need for medical staff to care for injured Vietnamese civilians. While the United States financed the initiative, the Korean government provided manpower during the war. My husband thought again this opportunity was a good chance for us to create the life that we had dreamed of. In Vietnam, a nurse's salary was $350 per month, plus an additional

IV—The Vietnam War

$100 housing allowance each month, compared to only $30 a month in South Korea. Plus, we would have access to the Post Exchange (PX) and could remain in touch, which had been the main way I'd communicated with Insok during his time in Vietnam. Yes, I agreed with Insok that this was a good idea, but I was hesitant. I was the mother of our daughter. If I were to die, then what would happen to my daughter? I suffered serious conflict about whether to go to Vietnam as a hospital nurse—after all, I hated working in the hospital. Most important, I didn't want to leave my baby girl behind with my mother-in-law, although she was a lovely person. But since we had many debts, we were looking for a chance like this to get our heads above water once again. Further, we could buy a house, which was an impossible dream for us at that time. I recalled my promise to myself before I married my husband: There is nothing love cannot face; there is no limit to its faith, its hope, its endurance (1 Corinthians 13:7).

But I had to think of my daughter's future. If I died on the battlefield in Vietnam, then my daughter's life would be worse than my own, which had been so harsh and tough, full of suffering. Sadly, from a cultural perspective, being an orphan in Korea was seen as shameful, leading to a life of misery. Her life would be much worse than mine. And I hoped that my daughter would never ever be hungry, disrespected, miserable, or sad. The more I thought about my daughter, the more I was in anguish. What I had heard about the war in Vietnam was that it was very different from the traditional way of war in the past. The chance of survival could be half that of other wars. It was called the "Vietcong War," which meant they did not care about the time and place. Fighting could happen at any time and anywhere, like at home, on the streets, at the market, in the fields, and so on. Simply, they did not have any uniform or boundaries or sense of day and night, not even seasons. Even among the crowds, it was hard to distinguish who was who. The risk would be great, but the money from joining the war effort would save us.

I was in deep contemplation again like when I was in high school, with no help from others. As a man, the first son in Korean culture, Insok had more responsibilities when it came to supporting our new home. I had to decide by myself what I would do. If I were to die, then I would die for the love of the family. As we had promised to each other,

From North Korea to America Through Three Wars

"There is nothing love cannot face." To live and conquer poverty, I had to do something unusual, something that required a great risk and bravery. I decided to go for the money, not to care for others like the famous nurse Florence Nightingale during the Crimean War in October 1854.

Up until this point, I had been brave and worked diligently to lift my family out of poverty and rid ourselves of the debts that haunted us. But then suddenly, I wondered again why all these terrible things kept happening to me. I relived my life since crossing the DMZ, and forgotten and hidden old memories and horrors resurfaced. That feeling of despair and defeat overwhelmed me. At night, I pondered that there must be no God. I cried hard and was full of sorrow. It felt as though everything I had done to better my life did not matter. There was no one I could ask for help again, of course not my brother due to his objection, but the reality stood in front of me, insurmountable. The only thing I had was unlimited love for my family. And my life never allowed me to rest or be at peace anyway, nor find help or counsel. It all seemed like fate, never free will. I was standing in between fate and love. I decided to go to Vietnam to fight for a better future out of love for my daughter, and I finally understood the love my mother had for us and felt the same drive that she must have felt since we left Daegwon-dong. My daughter was about two years old, and my mother-in-law would take care of her, but I remained in deep anguish. I held my daughter, hoping that she would not become an orphan in her life. She did not know why I was crying so hard while I was hugging her at Gimpo Airport in Seoul. Young Kyu and I cried nonstop as my daughter did not understand why, but the time came for me to go with the medical team to Vietnam. I left my beloved child in the arms of my mother-in-law and said goodbye, possibly for the last time.

The medical team had been organized by the Korean government, which included medical doctors, internists, surgeons, nurses with more than two years of experience in nursing, X-ray and lab technicians, and administrators for a one-year extendable contract in Vietnam. There were many different teams depending on geography. Each team had different numbers of staff according to need. The government called each team when it was time to board an airplane as a group. When I got the call, I left for Vietnam with tears in my eyes. My

IV—The Vietnam War

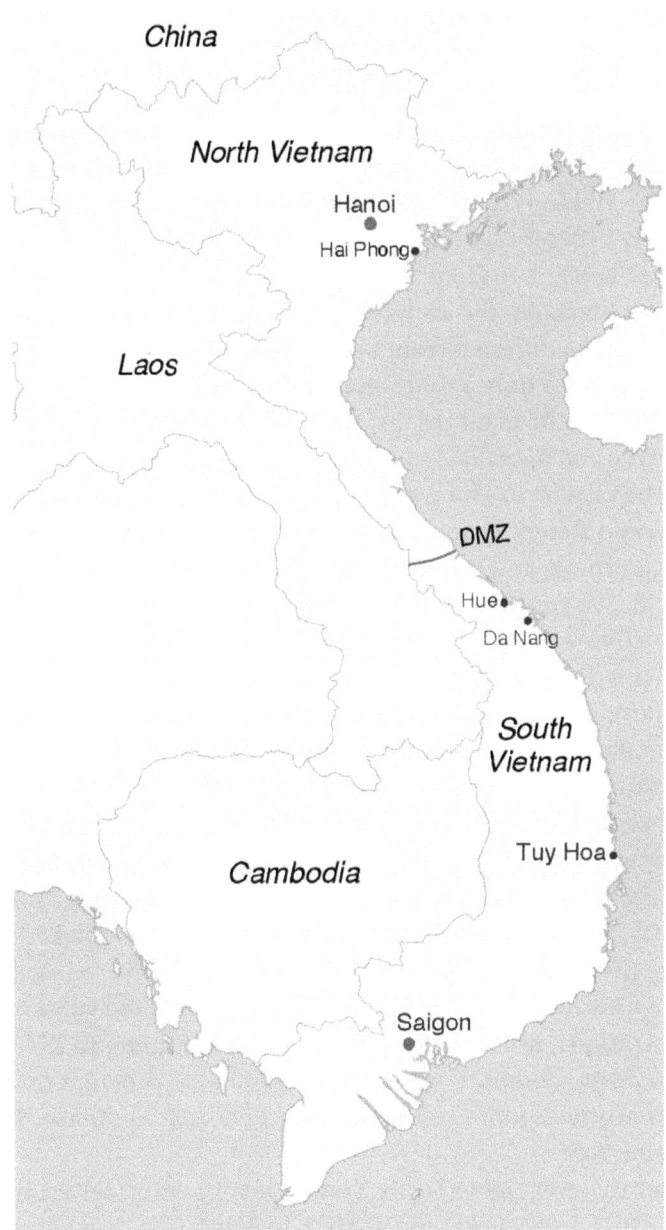

Map of Vietnam during the war in Vietnam. Outline map of Vietnam, ASEANUP, https://aseanup.com/free-maps-asean-countries/, with modifications (all wording and DMZ line) by Tisha S. Woo.

team flew from Seoul late one afternoon, with a layover scheduled in Hong Kong. It was the first time that I took an airplane, but I was neither excited nor curious. My mind was only occupied by my daughter who did not know why I had to leave her. It was night when we landed at Hong Kong airport—the sight of the city below was magnificent, with all kinds of lights that I had never even imagined. It was a completely different world, and I understood immediately why people wanted to come to Hong Kong to see this luxurious city, the stores, the women's fashion, the architecture (it was my first time seeing skyscrapers!), all so different from Seoul. The sight was breathtaking, but I could enjoy it for only a short moment because I missed my daughter. The more I saw the good things, the more I missed her. I felt that this was the true and natural love of mother to daughter.

At the airport in Hong Kong, we all were speechless. The airport looked very different from Seoul's. It was an international airport with enormous crowds and many colorful signs for departures and arrivals in English. We concentrated on our way through the airport because we were all new to these circumstances. I paid attention to not lose sight of the director of our team. I had a flashback to crossing the DMZ again. After I settled to wait for the boarding announcement, I saw the departure schedule in English to Los Angeles, New York, and Washington, D.C., for the first time in my life. I suddenly felt that there were two different worlds on earth: one was the battlefield and the other was peace. I realized I'd only ever found myself in war. I felt that I was too far away from those people who were going to L.A., New York, and D.C. Abruptly, I was afraid of dying. Then I asked myself, touching the railings, "Will I come back to touch this rail again?" My thoughts were heavy and intense, and again I wondered why I had endless frustrations, unlike other people who were going to L.A. Then I saw some team members, whose demeanors were different from mine and their attitudes more controlled, and I became less tense. We were in the same boat.

After the overnight stay in Hong Kong, the medical team left for Saigon, which today is known as Ho Chi Minh City. We boarded our flight. For how long we flew, I do not remember. I had no interest in looking out the window like others while flying to Saigon. Most of the time, I kept thinking about what I would do if something terrible

IV—The Vietnam War

happened to me. While I was ruminating over the future, I heard only one word over the speaker: "Saigon." I assumed that the pilot must have announced that we were approaching Saigon soon. So I looked out of the small window and saw all dark green jungles with no loose spaces between trees. It was the first time that I saw palm trees in my life. But the terrain scared me. It was a flat, endless dark green sea covered in patches of yellow dust. I imagined that no human could survive here; only animals like snakes and monkeys could live freely. The strange scene below made me realize that I was no longer home but in Vietnam, which scared me even more. I could only think of life and death. Without warning, I started to weep, but I discovered that my colleagues, who had the same feelings, were controlling them, unlike me. I had to control myself more than before because we, as a team, were all in the same situation. We all had families.

We landed at Saigon airport just before sunset and it was lightly raining. We had to walk from the plane to the gate because the pathway was not connected. While we were walking, we had to avoid craters from bombs. Seeing these holes blasted into the tarmac and hearing cannons, still so familiar, in the distance reminded me of the Korean War. No one needed to tell me that we were in Vietnam; war was everywhere around us, even before we checked in. After passing through customs, I saw a U.S. soldier sleeping on the floor in the middle of the hall, arms crossed, using his gun as a pillow. Under his body was nothing but the cement floor, yet he looked sound asleep despite the noise from the crowds. Seeing this soldier, I guessed that he was exhausted from the battlefield. Otherwise, how could he sleep among this crowd? Quickly, my old memories from the Korean War reminded me that I had to be alert and know what to do in this circumstance. I remembered how to live in a war again.

After a while, our guide arrived. We had some instruction on the current situation and what we had to do as medics in Vietnam. Before I was transferred to Tuy Hoa, located to the north, far from Saigon, I visited the market, curious to explore downtown. It was jarring to see the people act so worry-free despite the war. Everyone was busy shopping in the marketplaces, buying vegetables, merchandise, suits, and lingerie from France, as if life were completely normal. For a moment, despite there being no skyscrapers or magnificent lights, it felt no

From North Korea to America Through Three Wars

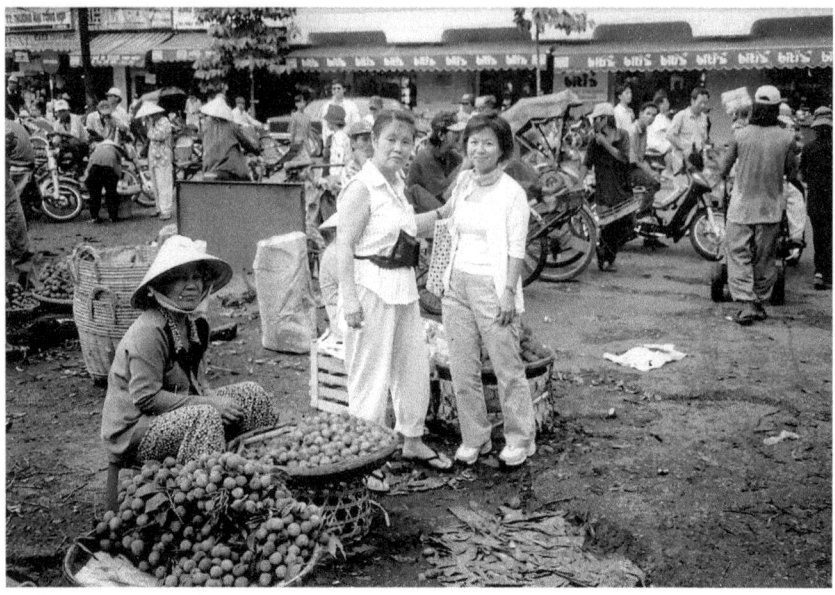

Sung Yoo (center, with black belt) on her first visit to a Vietnamese market after arriving in Saigon, 1968.

different than Hong Kong. I had never expected to see these beautiful things in Vietnam. Immediately, while the boom of nonstop cannon fire raged in the distance, I wondered how the people even cared about such luxuries during the war. I was floored; I was the only person who seemed to realize that there was a war going on all around. Then I wondered what kind of war was this? Was it even true that Vietnam was at war? During the war in Korea, we struggled immensely, and there were no nice things to buy at the markets. The experience was resoundingly different. But soon I spotted American soldiers with guns on their shoulders in the crowds. It was strangely comforting and not scary like the Korean War. Naturally, I wanted to buy these beautiful things when I saw them, but under temptation, I remembered that I was there to make money. Sometimes gunshots sounded off near to where I was, but the people seemed to not take notice. By chance, the medical team and I stumbled upon a tearoom, discovering many U.S. soldiers and Vietnamese girls wearing magnificent dresses and playing violins. It looked like they were having a party. There was ice cream in five different colors in a glass dish—I never knew there were so

IV—The Vietnam War

many flavors and that ice cream could be so beautiful. Unable to speak Vietnamese and knowing only broken English, we ordered ice cream, which a waitress brought to us in a big bowl. The ice cream looked so fancy; it was almost uncomfortable to eat. I was so surprised and hesitant to eat because I was in awe. We asked each other, "Where are we?" We could not believe we were in a war zone.

Ultimately, I arrived at my assigned civilian residence in Tuy Hoa with two other nurses. The head nurse, surgical nurses, and anesthesia nurse had arrived before us and could tell us what to do. At the hospital, we wore our nursing uniform, but while at home, we donned black pants and a white shirt like Vietnamese women, along with a traditional Vietnamese hat. When I arrived on the first day, it was midnight, and I felt like everything was new to me. Suddenly, before I went to sleep, I heard gunshots, and it felt like the gunman was standing right outside the door to the house. I feared he would try to enter the house, gun drawn. The head nurse switched off the light and told us not to talk, scream, or cry but to grab our passports and be ready to run in case the fighting got dangerously closer. Having a passport would be the only way I could escape Vietnam were something to happen. We sat on the floor in silence, scared to death, while gunfire erupted in the distance. It was terrifying to hear nonstop gunshots so close. We all sat in the dark room without knowing where to go, what to do, or how long it would last. We just breathed, remaining motionless, until dawn. At that moment, I felt that I'd made a big mistake coming to Vietnam. Even though I was afraid, I did not pray to God and Jesus for help because at that time, I no longer believed in them. Although I wasn't invincible, I only had faith in myself. I kept thinking and asking if this was the reason why we, the civilian nurses in Vietnam, got paid so well. I wondered what would happen if I were killed by the gunmen—I would leave my daughter behind as an orphan. This gunshot was like what I used to hear during the Korean War but not this close and strong at night near the houses. I sensed that immediately this was a big indication of guerrilla war, which meant that it could happen anywhere and anytime. We did not know how long the fighting lasted, but the sounds grew a little softer when dawn came. I went out to see if there were any bodies lying in front of the house, but there was nothing there. Since we were not used to hearing those sounds, I initially thought the fighting had happened right outside. Later, we found out that there had been a Vietcong attack several blocks away from where we were. That was why the gunfire sounds felt so strong and close.

The morning came and I went to the hospital for the first time with the other nurses, escorted by a Vietnamese driver. The moment I arrived at the hospital, I saw many traumatized people from last night's attacks crowded together, crying and mourning in Vietnamese. Before us, there were Vietnamese nurses who were instructing them and trying to organize who should have surgeries and treatment depending on the injuries sustained. Inside the hospital, various injured Vietnamese people were waiting for our teams, especially the surgeons. Before I got to know the hospital, I had to provide care depending on priority: gunshots, bleeding, skin tears, and big or small injuries. I felt that this really reminded me that I was in the war zone, although I did not see any soldiers in uniforms with guns; instead, it was "guerrilla" warfare. They were all civilians: old and young, men and women, and children as well. The men and women usually wore long black pants and shirts, but some of the men were in short pants

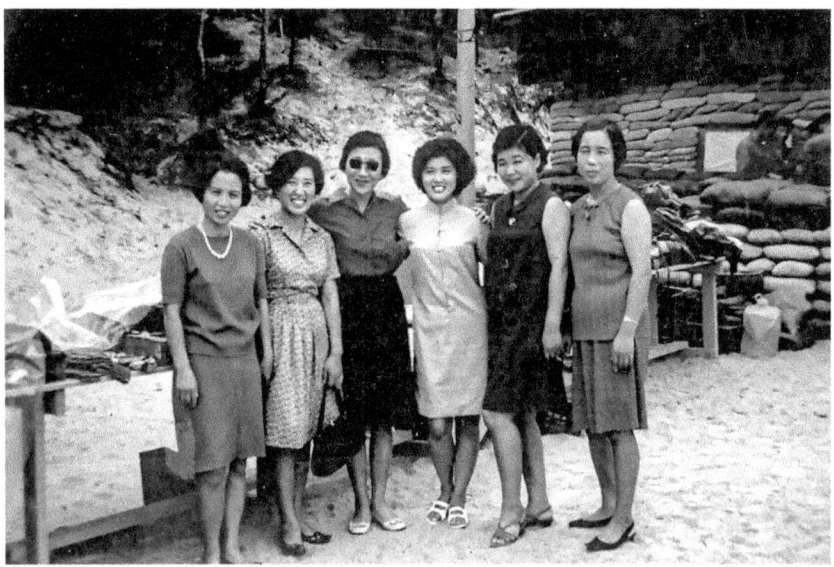

The Korean civilian medical team in Tuy Hoa, Vietnam, fall 1968. Sung Yoo is fourth from left.

IV—The Vietnam War

and plastic sandals only. The people were not bigger than us; rather, they were thinner, smaller than Koreans. But they scared me since the soldiers didn't wear uniforms; I couldn't distinguish between the Vietcong and civilians. Inside the operating room, it was cool thanks to the air conditioner, but the electricity was unreliable. When the power went out, generators would kick on. The heat, in general, was very different between the sun and shade: under the direct sun, it was unbearable, but under trees or shades or inside the house, it was tolerable. I understood why the people wore bamboo hats. The hospital was sturdily built originally by the French before the war, but there'd been little maintenance or upkeep due to the fighting. The beds were simple, just a bamboo mat. There was never enough water to clean the floor, which was mostly cement and tiles. The sanitary conditions were so poor, with flies and insects in the patient rooms and no air-conditioning except in the operating room. People did not care about the bugs, but they bothered me.

When I saw the patients, I felt so sad for them; they had been living through war for a long time and appeared tired and worn out. They were mute and rarely smiled at me. I had deep sympathy for their lives, but I was unable to talk to or share this with them at all because of the language barrier. My mind was full of understanding of their terrible situation and feelings about the war. It was hard not communicating with them, but I pretended that I had nothing to say and swallowed my feelings. At this point, I felt that I was helpless not sharing with them my compassion for their agonies because I, too, had my own experiences being in war.

But I had some observations that they were not the same as Koreans when we had the war. Surprisingly, their daily lives did not show their pain or sadness until tragedy struck. They wore very simple clothes: females wore black long pants with a white shirt and always the traditional hat, while males wore short pants that looked like underwear and sandals. When driving their motorcycles or riding their bikes, regardless of gender, both men and women wore black sunglasses, and some females wore ao dai with long black gloves, which looked very romantic.

The Vietnamese seemingly did not show any appreciation for getting help from Koreans or Americans. I did not observe any worry or fear of the cannon fire or gunshots, which boomed in the distance like in Saigon. Again, no one seemed to pay any attention. While I jumped from the sounds in the distance, the Vietnamese had no reaction—I couldn't tell if they were dull or *bali bali*, a Korean word meaning "hurry hurry" that speaks to Korean attitudes toward working hard, moving quickly, and hustling in daily life. But I concluded that they were numb because war had been routine, and they were used to it.

Vietnamese nurses worked hard, and they acted as junior physicians, doing sutures without a doctor's order. Although their nursing education level was no higher than the Koreans, we were not allowed to perform such duties. I learned from the Vietnamese nurses that they were trained in nursing skills by the French, learning from a different BSN curriculum than we Korean nurses. But we Korean nurses had good relationships with the Vietnamese. And they appreciated us for our care, although we did not speak their language. They tried to be cooperative with us when it came to language and cultural differences. Historically, the Vietnamese had an opportunity to have Chinese cultural customs a long time ago, so some Vietnamese were able to read Chinese characters as well as understand Confucianism and respect for the elderly. Additionally, Vietnamese culture had been influenced by the French. For that reason, I had to learn it and say it as they did. The Vietnamese said "merci beaucoup" commonly and naturally as a daily word. I had the chance to carry on a conversation with a male college student, who was a sophomore at Saigon University but had taken a year off due to a physical condition. He explained to me that in high school, he read a few novels in French, and he could speak better French than English. He dreamed of studying in Paris, but due to the war, he was unable to travel to France. While he carried on the conversation with me, he used French words often.

Most of their houses were built in the French style with fancy gardens, and I often forgot that I was still in Asia because the homes looked so different from ours in Korea and those in Japan. Even though most of the houses were run-down or destroyed because of the fighting, I felt like I could imagine the people inside living wonderful lives. And I imagined going to France and seeing these same homes and gardens maybe lining the streets of Paris.

One night while we were sleeping, a Vietnamese driver came to us

IV—The Vietnam War

in a hurry and reported an attack by the Vietcong in a nearby village. All the villagers were at the hospital with injuries. As soon as we heard the news, we all rushed to the hospital in his car. When we arrived, there were people everywhere, old and young, men and women, crying mothers and children. The Vietnamese nurses had arrived before us. Our priority was those with more serious injuries, and I remember one of my patients was a young man in a black shirt and pants on a stretcher, who was being followed by his wife. She cradled her younger child, who was no more than eight months, while her older child stood on her left side, holding her hand. I checked her husband's vital signs but couldn't read any. Then I immediately reported that he had no vital signs to a Vietnamese nurse, and she informed his wife. The wife was speechless, and her skin turned white as she looked down at her husband on the stretcher. Then she looked at her baby in her arms, whose head dropped forward lifelessly. She shook the baby again and again but did not get any response. She did not know what she had to do at that time, between her husband's and baby's deaths. We, the nurses, doctors, and other medics, all froze and couldn't speak to her, not because of the language barrier but because we knew what had happened. In silence, we exchanged looks, unable to formulate words, but our expressions reflected how we felt deep in our hearts. Our eyes became like birds' eyes "signaling about these deaths." We saw, but we acted like we did not see this death because our eyes couldn't move. The woman of tragedy was mute and white on her face like a dead body. She did not move while holding her dead baby. This was the worst tragedy that I had ever seen in my life. This was the most lamentable scene, with the sudden deaths of her husband and her child at the same time, in the same place, and in front of her. Who could say a word? Suddenly, our compassion covered her, and we asked for her, "What was the war for?" "Why?" We all cried for her with tears in our hearts, regardless of whether we were Vietnamese or Korean, since we were all human beings.

I wanted to have this whole scene burned into my memory because the thing could not be explained. Nevertheless, the scene remained as a rock because it couldn't be burned. The memory remained as fresh as vegetables after a summer rain.

Not long after the first attack, there was another at night in the village about one hour away from the hospital. Under the command of our team's leader, we all went to the village by car and saw the scene, what had happened at night into the early morning. Houses were still on fire—smoldering and wheezing—and the villagers wept, sitting in the dirt. We were busy helping the injured and spending time comforting the people. According to the villagers, the Vietcong had arrived that previous night and dragged away young men by force. Then they set the houses ablaze and fled. The remaining villagers were mainly the elderly and young children. Our team was trying to attend to their medical needs and put out the fires as much as we could. On that day, I clearly remember one old lady wearing black pants and a shirt with a white cap, sitting on the ground by the rice paddies, crying in Vietnamese. Of course, I could not understand a word, but I sensed that why she was crying and talking to herself was because of her sorrow. She felt completely lost and helpless. The way she cried reminded me of when I was desperate and helpless in the past and of my mother crying, too. Naturally, I cried as well, seeing her there, unable to speak to her but understanding from the heart, nevertheless. At this moment, I was aware that we human beings had no need to speak of our sorrows or tragedy verbally. Our hearts were enough to talk together in sorrow.

I didn't have a sense of time in Vietnam, and memories pop into my head. I remember making rounds at the hospital one day, observing one young Vietnamese man wearing only short pants, who was chained to his bamboo bed by one leg. In his early twenties, he didn't appear to be anxious or in pain, but rather, he was halfway smiling when he saw me. I greeted him in Vietnamese, "How are you?" and he responded the same to me as well. I noticed that he had heavy dressing on the lower portion of his unshackled leg, which he couldn't and shouldn't move. Through his medical record, I found out that he was a Vietcong soldier who fought all night in the rice paddies and had been shot in his lower right leg. After being injured, he was unable to run away fast enough and was caught by a South Vietnamese soldier. Since he was captured nearby, he was brought to the civilian hospital where I worked until he could be transferred to the army hospital. The Vietnamese nurse explained to me that the Vietcong spirit was strong, and they will keep running until they fall over. I thought that he was brave as a soldier despite being communist. While he was with

IV—The Vietnam War

us, he was not discriminated against. He was just another patient on the floor who deserved the same care as everyone else. He did not act any different, like an enemy, and the Vietnamese nurses were naturally kind to him. In this situation, I learned from these Vietnamese nurses to treat all lives as equal. Instinctively, I remembered my experience back when I came to South Korea in 1948. At that time, I wanted to have this kind of kindness. But instead of kindness, I was discriminated against for being a refugee from the North Korea. Through this observation, I sensed that the Vietnamese were more open minded. Despite Vietnam and South Korea both being in Asia, the Vietnamese had a different attitude toward those who had a different ideology. I felt that this was a good opportunity to compare the characters of two different countries in the same continent of Asia. The attitude was not the same. I wondered what the causes were that made them different. Were they somehow related to the perspectives of religion, history, or geographic location? Finally, I wondered how these Vietnamese character traits, so different from the Koreans', had persisted even after having been at war with each other for so long.

I kept thinking about this observation ever since: Why is the culture so different between Vietnam and Korea? If we could understand the reasons, then it would be nice for generations yet to come. I wished I had been able to study based on my interest or observations.

Then again, I had a question about the war: Why did we fight among ourselves in one nation between north and south, like Korea and Vietnam? Of course, it was due to the difference in ideology between communism and democracy. And my family is one of the many victims of this fight. Then this thought led me to continue to think of the Vietnamese woman who had lost her husband and baby at the same time in front of me and her at the hospital. Then suddenly, I looked at recalling about the democracy that was deeply related to the current situation where I was. I realized I had been in two real battlefields seeing this tragedy—Korea and Vietnam—not as a soldier but as a civilian, as a child in Korea and as a nurse in Vietnam when I was in my late 20s. What should I do because of experiencing and seeing these tragedies? Should I become a war historian or psychologist? I felt that I had some responsibility to make the difference for the future with sorrow, frustration, and tragedies. My thoughts of pains and agonies became deeper and bitter, but after a while, I realized why I came to Vietnam. At one point through this thought process, I came to have a feeling, which was very important, of humanity. This feeling was applied to everyone regardless of nationality sincerely from my heart.

I wished that I could speak Vietnamese so that I could at least have consoled her and shared my own experiences growing up during war. I could show her that she was not alone. She shouldn't give up hope because I was in a similar situation. But I could not do anything. There was nothing I could do for her, unlike my mind, which made me sadder. I felt like I was lost in dark tunnels with neither light nor food. I was alone and helpless in the dark. But the reality woke me up, reminding me that I needed to make some money for my own lovely daughter and family. Then my hope and love asked me what I had to fight for survival for myself and all my family as I promised. My tough reality made me go on into the real world.

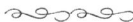

I recalled the real world when I went to the PX for my daily things. Like when I was in Saigon, I was shocked to see all the groceries and merchandise the Americans had in Vietnam, stored in a building the size of a Whole Foods. Each section had different items like Macy's, but what was most surprising was seeing mink coats, shawls, and collars. I bought some of the collars. I also purchased a Japanese pearl necklace, Mikimoto brand, which was known to be famous and expensive. That's how I learned the name of pearls, from Mikimoto. Another surprise was buying an entire Noritake china set, which was also famously known as good porcelain, Western-style, and charming. All these made me open my eyes to a modern lifestyle from the battlefield. Also, I was impressed to see Johnnie Walker Scotch whisky: big bottles and small bottles lined up on a wall, from top to bottom, viewed as an expensive present for fancy people. As soon as I saw them, my mouth opened widely, and I asked the person next to me, "Did I see the name Johnnie Walker correctly?" The answer was "Yes." Those unimaginable bottles made me once again ask the same question, "Who drinks whisky in the battlefield?" Then I saw a Morton salt container, 26 oz for only 5 cents, making me light up. When I

IV—The Vietnam War

saw this salt, I sensed that America was truly different from Korea and Vietnam because I had never thought of selling salt in a paper container with a fixed price. Often, in Korea, such merchandise was bargained for in the markets. To see and observe the things in the PX, I felt that I was near to America. I could imagine why people wanted to move to America, which further inspired me to go there. This was an unexpected but eye-opening opportunity for me because I had come to Vietnam during war. With this recognition, for the first time, I felt that my decision to come to Vietnam was right.

Much later, Insok was moved from Saigon to join me through his company, which was unique and rare for a couple together during the war. Even though I was reunited with my husband, I still had the same feelings of missing my daughter more than ever because I wanted to share with her everything that had happened, the good and the bad. I discovered that this kind of feeling was a mother's love. But I had to hide the feelings inside because other nurses, who were all mothers like me, had their husbands. I assumed they had the same feelings I had. During that encounter with Insok, we convened in the meeting room for families at war. It was available 24/7 to anyone seeking to reunite with their spouse since families were understandably not allowed in the battlefield. The room had a slate roof and was open on three sides but protected with mosquito nets. There was always classical music playing to console and soothe guests.

One day, a high-ranking Korean officer of the White Horse unit who was stationed not far from Tuy Hoa, wanted to taste Korean barbecue, so he sent a big box of T-bone steak to Insok and me. I had never seen that meat before. I'd never expected to see that much beef in my life, nor did I know that meat existed in the shape of a "T." The meat came in a huge box from the United States for soldiers. I didn't know that meat could be stored this way, frozen, and kept so fresh. Seeing and touching the steak, I wondered how much it cost and admired the skilled, scientific way it was cut. Again, I couldn't believe that this was delivered from the States to my hands in a war zone in hot weather. It was another instance of how Americans seemed much more advanced. Their butchering skills indicated how advanced Americans were in handling foods. I admired the way they did it. Immediately, I recalled how the Korean soldiers were treated during the Korean War almost

From North Korea to America Through Three Wars

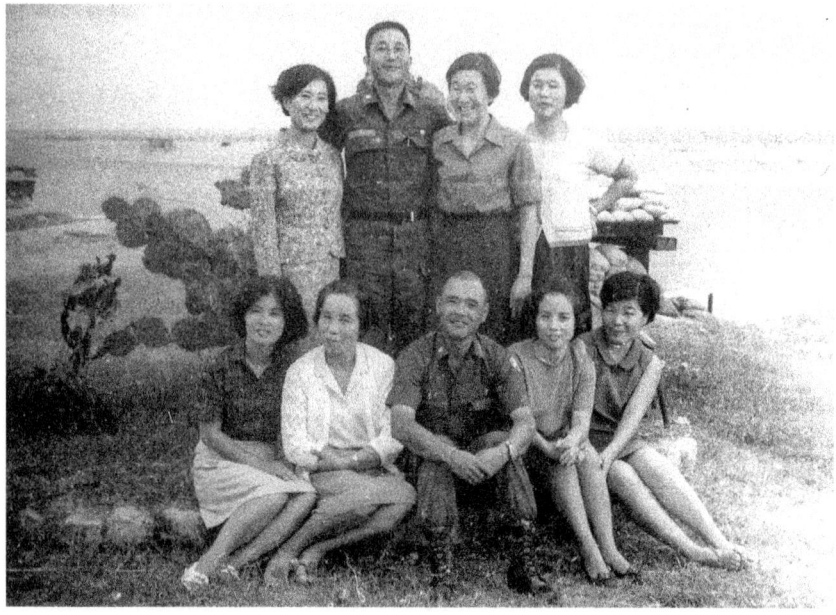

Sung Yoo (front row, at left) with other Korean civilian medical team nurses at a White Horse Division station with two Korean officers, late 1968.

a decade ago. I saw what they were eating when they escaped from the place where my family used to live in Nusang-dong in Seoul in 1950. There was no comparison between what the American soldiers ate and what the Korean soldiers ate in the battlefield.

All the Korean nurses knew how to cook traditional Korean barbecue, but we had several problems, including not having enough utensils or big bowls and access to only a very small kitchen in hot weather with no charcoal, no grill, etc. We barely had ingredients like green onions, Vietnamese soy sauce, garlic, and sesame seed oil. However, it turned out well, and everyone had a good time eating the T-bone. The officer who brought the steak was not only happy with the meal but excited to see females again because he missed his wife as well. He even brought a big can of shrimp, which was so expensive in the land of America. Again, I had never seen these fresh large shrimps which were kept for a long time in the can. My husband and I tried to console the medical team members by sharing the feast with them as

IV—The Vietnam War

one big family because they missed their spouses at home. Even my husband's coworkers joined in on the feast, and one on his colleagues bought me a Rolex watch because he missed his wife and was happy that Insok got to see me. It felt like he was seeing his own wife, he said.

Approaching the end of the year, I heard that the Korean medical team had been invited to a Christmas party by the U.S. soldiers who were stationed nearby in the jungle. When I heard about this party invitation, I was not glad at all because my mind was occupied with fear of the present circumstances, from the sounds of cannons and guns to missing and worrying about my two-year-old daughter back home in Korea. But I realized that as part of a team, I had to move along with them.

For the party, they asked us to wear customary Korean clothing, which we were told to bring before we left for Vietnam. It looked awkward to me in this situation, but we all wore it. We traveled together in one car, nervous and curious about attending a party with Americans, especially soldiers, on the battlefield, which was entirely new to me. I do not remember how long it took to get there, but I was able to sense that the scenery was becoming deeper, quieter, and darker. It looked as if no human being could possibly exist in this environment. But the car kept going. As we approached the army base, I could see only jungle: big trees with no space, vines, and dark green woods. But I was able to see the battle bunker, which was surrounded by heavy, dark green sandbags, cannons, and guards, all standing like chopsticks with eyes like the rays from the sun. This scene was quite opposite from Saigon or Tuy Hoa, and finally I felt that I was in the real battlefield.

One U.S. soldier came to us and led us to the party room. As soon as we entered, I was stunned and almost lost my mind because it was a completely different world. The room was bright and joyful and adorned with Christmas decorations: Christmas trees in silver, green and red socks hung here and there, and there were colorful candies everywhere. Even more exhilarating were the Christmas carols: "O Holy Night," "White Christmas," "Silent Night," and so on. Seeing and listening, I was overwhelmed by the unexpected things all around me. I was lost, unable to decide what I should look at or do or listen to. Of course, my English was in no way conversational. Only the wondering existed. However, I immediately felt that all the fear, anxiety, and worry were gone. I forgot all the agonies, worries, and fears. It was unbelievable things happened.

The most surprising moment was an invitation to dance from an American, who was double the size of me. I was astonished and motionless, unable to talk even. I did not know what to do. Never had I been asked to dance by a stranger, not even in Korea. I wasn't expecting this invitation at all. I felt that he sensed that I was shocked, but he kept smiling at me. I gestured "No, thank you"; however, he once again gently insisted on dancing. To be nice, without a word, I stood up and followed him as he moved, with neither style nor form. Soon, I felt that he could not continue to dance with me anymore. He finally offered me a glass of orange juice and left. I was very much relieved since I was able to keep to myself as before.

Surprisingly, I was able to listen to carols, which brought me to remember my daughter at home and others in the past. I wished to be with my daughter. I looked at the people dancing and listening to carols, and I forgot all about the war outside, that I was in Vietnam. Suddenly, I felt like I was at home. I was comfortable. It was a good healing opportunity. I wanted this moment last forever, but it went away quickly.

Surprisingly, I hesitated to leave, but I knew that I must go. I thanked the American soldiers for the invitation, and I regretted the way how I initially understood the party. In fact, I began to understand why people wanted to celebrate and enjoy Christmas. It was comfort, a sense of peace, which we all wanted to experience at that party just for fun and joy. I learned from this party what was the meaning of "peace." After all, weren't we fighting for this peace in Vietnam and Korea? This unanswered question was deeply seated in my mind. It was a precious moment and joyful, but the minute I headed back outside, I was aware of the war again. Nevertheless, I felt different than before I entered the party. It was a good opportunity to understand what the meaning of party was. I really enjoyed and appreciated the invitation. It was my first time to be at a party like this.

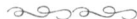

All Korean nurses were granted access to the Seventh Air Force Officer Club in Tuy Hoa, a city on the East Vietnam Sea that was home

IV—The Vietnam War

to an air force base. It was not far from where I resided. Although my English was not yet proficient, I visited the club along the sea out of curiosity to see how the Americans soldiers lived in Vietnam. When I entered the club, I immediately discovered that it was totally different than the jungle where I was for the Christmas party. Of course, it was by the sea, but the structure of the club was unimaginably clean, cool, and calm, with soft classical music playing. There were several officers who were lying down on the floor freely and sitting on the chair reading books, but no one talked or paid attention to who came and went. It looked silent and serene before the floor-to-ceiling window facing the sea. My eyes absorbed the scene. Through the glass wall, I was able to see the whole sea, quiet and tranquil, existing only in peace and brilliantly reflecting the sunlight. It was really comforting. I cannot recall how long I gazed at the sea before wondering what I should do at the club. It was decorated in a modern style with a piano, record player, and bookshelves. Wherever I looked, it was not the same scene that I used to see in Korea or Vietnam. I asked myself, "Am I in the right place?" No one paid attention to me. However, I stood for a while, still as a snowman. Enchanted by the sea, I was eventually approached by a soldier who offered me a drink. I answered, "No, thanks" because I was uncomfortable to speak to him in my broken English, but inside of me I had and wanted to talk a lot to share with him my feelings. At that time, whoever was in the room, the soldier left his mother, sister, wife, or fiancée for the nation, but I was there for the money. I felt guilty, but their duty was their country's protection. I found myself once again pondering why I existed, a question that stuck with me throughout my life and one that I still think about today.

I wished I was able to speak in English so that I could share with these soldiers my feelings and thoughts. These feelings inspired me to study English more than before. Many times, I felt that I needed to study English for my own good and improving my life like going to America. Sometimes, because of what I saw in Vietnam, I began to dream of going to America, but my reality was not simple yet. At that moment, I missed my daughter, and I suddenly saw the sea as an enemy because although it was strikingly beautiful, it was an obstacle to surmount to return home to my daughter. Realizing the present situation, I had two contrasting ideas of the sea: hate and love, beauty and fear. Hiding my complex feelings, before taking a chair in the fancy room, I left quietly and calmly in tears, missing my baby. I just hoped that one day I would be able to explain to my daughter about these feelings in Korean or English.

My contract was ending, and it was time for me to return to South Korea. I was elated that none of our team members had been injured or killed despite spending a year together on the frontier of life and death. Even more, we were all happy to be returning home under better financial conditions, which we hoped for desperately. I noticed that we, the medical team, all became so close like a family in such a short time, even though we did not know one another before at all. Now it seemed as though we'd known one another for a lifetime, as though we were family members. After we left, we kept in touch over the years, just like a family. We met up a few times when we were home and even had a party. All anxieties and fears flew away like the chaff, and our hearts were filled with full joy.

Thankfully, my husband and I left Vietnam together. During our time in Vietnam, we worried about what might happen to each other, but we were healthy and returned home alive and happy, preparing to pay off all debts from the wedding and buy a house as well. On the way back home in Hong Kong, where I was initially terrified of possibly dying in Vietnam, we shopped limitlessly for ourselves. It was a pleasure for us, a celebration of us both making it home safely. That was all combined with a joy and delight that I had never experienced until now. I wondered whether I deserved to have this much delight. We learned from this experience many things: being brave and being explorers in the battlefields, even while we were missing and worrying about our daughter at home.

When I arrived back home in Seoul, I was simply happy to see my daughter who had grown taller and was talking better for her age, with a great vocabulary. We hugged, shedding tears of happiness, of course. There was no word for how happy I was! I couldn't express my gratitude for my mother-in-law, who took good care of my daughter, her granddaughter. We were all simply grateful and satisfied. No more debts, no more poverty, and no more worrying that my daughter would become an orphan were things that we worried the most about day

IV—The Vietnam War

and night. Not only that, my husband and I soon welcomed our second daughter, Hyo Min, beautiful and healthy, simply a gift and a blessing to our family. We couldn't expect anything else more than these blessings. We just had a new life. I forgot all the struggles, frustrations, and agonies that I had been through in the past from North Korea to Vietnam. Plainly, I was a new person, and everything was good, but I had to think of our future. I wondered whether I still wanted to be a nurse at a hospital. Of course, I did not want to be a nurse, although I made money by the nursing job. But now, I wanted change. Many thoughts were heavy: Should I remain a nurse or study for a PhD in nursing to teach or even go back to school for a different subject?

Although I was very happy to be back in Korea, I found that the people often looked down on me because of my North Korean background and my choice of nursing as a profession. These reflected old cultural concepts, which I disliked. Also, psychologically and frankly, I did not want to stay in nursing in Korea unless my position was changed to a professor or office worker due to my new experiences and

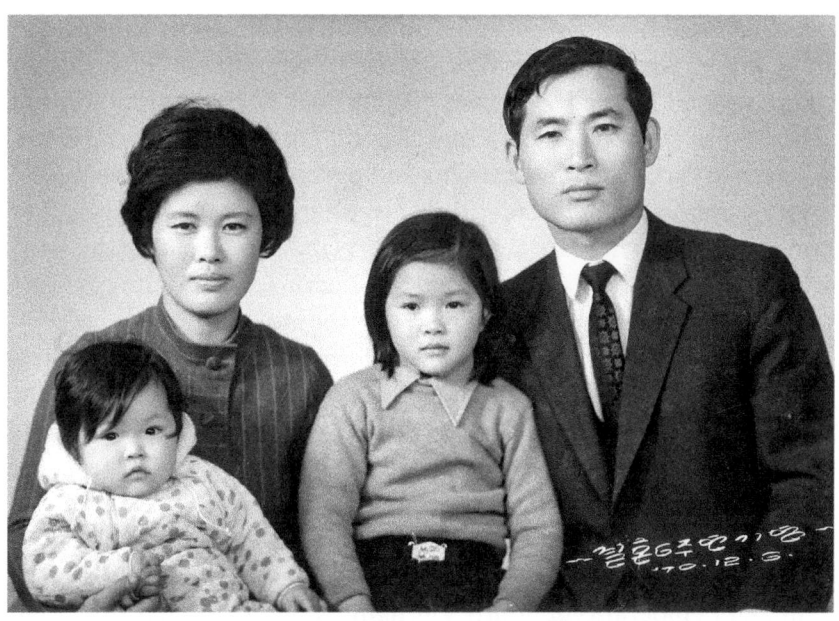

Family portrait Sung Yoo and Insok Yoo, with their children, Hyo Min (Peggy) and Hyen Ju (Julie), after their return from Vietnam.

knowledge from Vietnam. Frankly, I went to Vietnam to earn money, but unexpectedly, I learned much more than I thought I would.

There were cultural differences between Korea and Vietnam. The Vietnamese did not rush things. They did not keep daily life separate from the war and did not express appreciation for the help from Americans and Koreans. Of course, I did not ask every Vietnamese person questions about their feelings, but I did not hear often expressions of gratitude or facial expressions whenever they received any services or material things from Koreans or Americans. My sentiment was that they wanted to be "left alone." From this sense, often I had questioned how we Koreans had different attitudes and reactions during the Korean War. There were many other differences as well, but I was not able to sort them out.

I also began to discover many historical parallels between Vietnam and Korea. Vietnam was once owned by the French from the mid-19th century to the 1950s, which reminded me of Korea when we were under Japanese occupation from 1910 until 1945. We used Japanese words a lot in our daily conversations. Likewise, the Vietnamese used French words in their common conversations as well. For an example, they often easily used the French phrase "merci beaucoup," which I learned to say, for "Thank you." Many times, I was not able even to pronounce the French at all. On the roads, I often saw Western-style houses and gardens and parks that had been damaged severely by bombs, but I was still able to see the French influence. They said that Saigon (now Ho Chi Minh City) used to be called the Eastern Paris before the war. From this information, I had more curiosity to know about Vietnamese history with the stories and these scenes. Then I had a clue for the reasons why I saw the beautiful female lingerie at the market when I arrived in Saigon in 1968, even when the war was on. Also, in one tearoom there were five different colored ice-cream scoops in a beautiful glass dish. It was an amazing scene for me at that time.

Another identical aspect of political situations was the division of Vietnam into two parts like Korea: communist in North Vietnam and democratic in South Vietnam. When I realized this, I felt closer to the Vietnamese than before when I did not know. Although we used different languages, I guess we would share the same pain, sorrow, and problems emotionally and mentally. Learning about this unusual circumstance, my desire to learn more about politics and philosophy became stronger. Why did these unwanted situations happen on earth? This was another chance to open my eyes to the world with questioning, but there were no easy answers to that question either.

Besides learning these things, I had a very rare opportunity to live in a guerrilla war, something that I had heard about only in the news. Being in this war, I used to be afraid day and night because it was hard to figure out where it was safe and comfortable. Nobody knew who anybody was. Since they did not wear uniform, it was impossible to sense or figure it out. On the roads, everything looked normal. People were busy with their daily lives: eating, drinking, laughing, talking in their own languages, men and women, young and old, children running freely. People were riding bicycles or automobiles with dark sunglasses. I did not often see armies in uniforms of the Vietnamese or the Americans, but the civilians filled the road. For being in this war, I had learned many things, but the clearest thing was to be brave and alert.

Also, I had an opportunity to compare the characteristics of the war between the East (North Vietnam) and the West (the United States). While the Vietnamese had mental power formed by their religion of Buddhism, the United States had the power of technology of weapons and military powers: in other words, of the East versus the West. By these comparisons I had so many sad thoughts asking for what reasons this war was being fought. Another question regarded who the winner was of that war. Sadly, it was communism. That answer made me so sad because of my family and the experience of the Vietnamese woman who lost both her husband and her baby in a Vietcong attack. Is there any answer for that story? Don't I have a right to ask this question?

While I was in Vietnam, I hungered for cool air day and night. When I arrived in Seoul, I appreciated the cool air and realized how good it was. Yet I did not call for God, but I thought to myself, "I am lucky not to be dead."

V

Seeking the American Dream

As I'd dreamed for so long, we were all happy and healthy in our new house. The mood was like a long housewarming party, but our future was uncertain in the changed living conditions. I'd heard information from one of my friends that there was a shortage of nurses in the United States, and many Korean nurses were already going there since they dreamed of going to America, a known paradise in the world. The requirement for nurses was a nursing license and two years of experience in the nursing field. There was no need for an examination, in contrast to what was required for non-nurse students. It seemed impossible because many other students had to take such examinations to go to the States. So they studied hard, failing often. Understandably, whoever passed the examination was respected and admired by the people in general. In addition to not needing to take a test, nurses were also allowed to apply to go to the United States with their family, whereas students were not. With this information, I asked myself if this news could be true because when I applied to nursing school, my brother Sung Kul suggested that I go to America for a better future. At that time, a better future was in the air, too far away from me. I didn't think I'd ever be able to go. But then, I believed I could. I was unable to admit this thing, truly happening, as he advised me when I was in a dark time with no hope. This was absolutely, unexpectedly remarkable.

After I told Insok about this opportunity, he was highly delighted. He and I thought again about what we should do for our future and the children's education. He was so happy with this news—it was always his dream to go to America. Not knowing simply how hard it would

V—Seeking the American Dream

be to learn English and hospital work at the same time in the United States, I agreed with the idea, remembering how our employment in Vietnam ended up paying off. It would be another beginning for a better life. In this sense, I was thinking that if I did not go to America, what was going to happen to my family? The negatives of staying in South Korea as a nurse were outweighed by the positives of leaving. That gave me reason to go. In addition, we were able to afford tickets, which had not been possible before. Even though I could barely speak English, my husband was proficient enough to hold a conversation in the language.

Insok and I decided that my oldest daughter, who had just turned six, would come with us, while our younger daughter, who was only 18 months, would stay behind with my mother-in-law, Young Kyu. Bringing her along would make the transition more difficult because we would have to navigate finding a babysitter. We were not sure if we could take on the extra costs while figuring out life in another country. To fight for a better life, I once again had to leave a child behind. Of course, it was not like going to Vietnam, a matter of life and death, but leaving my child with Young Kyu, not hugging and loving her every day and knowing how much she would miss me would break my heart again. It was not that I did not trust my mother-in-law; we were getting along better than before, and I still appreciated all her help. Even though I wasn't leaving my daughter to go to a war zone, the feeling of hurt and misery were nevertheless the same. I became so emotional when it came time to depart for the United States. While I was hoping for a better life, I had to endure deep agonies, leaving a child two times, unlike the other mothers. This agony contrasted dramatically with the joyful reunion with my daughter after my return from Vietnam. But my past sufferings had given me the ability to act bravely and with endurance. Then I said to myself that I didn't want to be a dependent woman, as a traditional wife who was dependent on her husband. I wanted to face the challenges for a better life continuously.

But it was not easy to ignore these hardships as a mother being in this situation, expecting how much we will miss each other, not being able to lay my eyes on my daughter or hold her. It was bitter, painful, and sorrowful, but I had to stand against all obstacles. Pretending like

From North Korea to America Through Three Wars

I was ready to go to war again, I kept all my emotions inside of me. My heart became thick and heavy. I breastfed my daughter until it was time to go because I hoped to give her my touch and love as long as I could. When I was on the airplane, breast milk soaked through my dress and I started to cry, no matter how much I had determined to be strong. It was pure and natural, but I was embarrassed and crossed my arms over my breasts. I missed my baby. I imagined how much my baby wanted this milk to satisfy her hunger. That made me cry and cry until my tears dried. This memory has never faded away. It was beyond a mother's love: pure, natural, and innocent. Immediately, my old memories from Vietnam came back to me, how I missed my daughter in Tuy Hoa during the war. Then, again, I asked about my fate or doom, why my life wasn't the same as other women. But there was no answer, only full tears inside my heart. Unable to control myself, I kept crying with my older daughter, who was sitting next to me. She knew and missed her younger sister, too. At that time, I had continuously repeated the same questions to which there was no answer. I realized that I needed to persevere and swallow all the ulcerous agonies again. Nevertheless, I imagined how much my baby would cry looking for my breast milk. My mind ruminated over all this despair and agonies: Do I need to have more pain yet? Or forever? Was I born to live in this condition? Didn't I deserve to have joy or fortune after the Vietnam War? I forgot all my determinations that I made for coming to the United States, but I drowned into deep water.

Since I'd been born in North Korea, I saw Korean history unfold, which had become history. I realized quickly that I had been through three wars from my young age: World War II, the Korean War, and the Vietnam War. After World War II, all Koreans were so happy with the liberation from Japan, who had occupied Korea for 36 years. But shortly thereafter, whoever had been born in the North like me ended up suffering an arduous life. I'd never gotten to enjoy the normal life as teenage girls should. I had to live as a grown up too early, with sufferings, agonies, and pain, unable to dream. No one ever guided me as to how to live. I just jumped to be a grown-up adult with no help and little knowledge. I did not want my daughters to have such a life. Never. I had to be brave and resilient again. Soon, I saw my older daughter next to me, who deserved a better life. I pretended quickly that I had only

V—Seeking the American Dream

hope. But inside of me, I discovered that pretending to rely on hope was not easy.

As the plane landed in Seattle, Washington, on October 17, 1971, I looked out at the houses in neat lines and rows like cubes of tofu, the style so different from homes in Korea and Vietnam. I said to my husband, "Look how strange these homes are." Of course, the people spoke English, most of which I could not understand at all, so naturally I was completely dependent on my husband for everything inside Seattle airport, from using the bathroom to ordering tea. After a short layover, we arrived at the international airport in Washington, D.C. One of our relatives, my husband's uncle, came to meet us and led us to his apartment at 2:00 a.m. in Takoma Park, Maryland. He'd emigrated to the United States to obtain his PhD in political science and stayed after his studies. Insok and his uncle remained close even though they lived on different continents. The stories he told Insok about America had inspired my husband to want to move there. We were exhausted after traveling, but Insok's uncle was so excited to have us. When I woke up that morning, my eyesight was full of many tall trees, unlike the palm trees in Vietnam, which opened to a high, clean, blue sky. But on the inside, my mind was filled with my baby crying and looking for mom. At that moment, my breasts were full of milk for my younger daughter again. I felt that I wanted to run and grab my baby, but it was impossible. If I had been allowed to go back home, I would have gladly said "yes." Once more, I felt pure mother's love. But I had to remind myself that my new life in America would be better through endurance and patience. I forced myself to adjust to whatever I had to do. But it was worse with milk on my chest. Whereas the milk lasted about a week, the yearning to hold my baby once again never left.

Finally, I found a job as a graduate nurse—meaning, before I obtained an RN license in the States—on the Med-Surgical Unit of Providence Hospital in Washington, D.C. According to state law, any nurse who worked at a hospital in this country needed to be licensed in the United States, but I just had my Korean nursing license. In that sense, the hospital allowed me to work as a graduate nurse like an RN while I studied to complete my state board nursing examination. I was hired to work on this unit, which required speaking in English, as was having nursing clinical experiences in surgical and medical units. I was filled with anxiety because I knew that I had lacked English fluency and enough clinical experience at a hospital. Since the hospital needed nurses badly due to shortage of nurses at that time, they hired me. Nobody knew how to test the English level of new nurses because it had never happened in the past in the United States. It was a big challenge to both parties, foreign nurses and the hospitals.

Soon I learned that I was not in the right place to be hired, but I had to be there because other Korean nurses had almost the same problems. The amount of fear and worry was almost like the battlefield, but nobody knew how to handle and teach in this huge, scary, and unmeasurable situation. There was no orientation or class for solving problems like this. I just had to adjust to the situation by seeing or following the other American nurses. Even I was unable to describe how to do and what to do with these worries and fears. The language barrier faced me from the beginning when I had an interview with the nursing director on the first day, but surprisingly, I was hired.

Without knowing how to adjust, I felt suffocated by all these difficulties. I did not know where I should begin to learn the language and study for the examination. I'd never used an English textbook in Korea, only a few pamphlets in English depending on the subject and professor who had been in the United States for a short visit. I didn't even know there were five subject areas of the nursing textbook, each of which I had to take separately for the state examination. All the sudden changed circumstances, including the demands of English, became very heavy to bear, from beginning to the end. I needed to learn English to read and communicate at work, along with new nursing skills and knowledge. Since I did not know how to buy these textbooks, Insok had to do for me everything that I needed. While all other Korean nurses with clinical experiences struggled with English, my situation was worse than the other Korean nurses because of a lack of clinical experience. With all this on my mind, I worked extremely hard and almost didn't even have time to miss my daughter. My determination for a better life became stronger than before with all these newfound difficulties. I pushed myself, knowing that I had to overcome all these obstacles to achieve this long-awaited hope of a good life for my family. It was like during the war but without cannon fire and gunfire in the distance. I needed to persevere and force myself to

V—Seeking the American Dream

endure these hardships to bring my baby to the States as soon as possible. On the other hand, sometimes, when I was extremely tired, I asked myself if I weren't a nurse, would I still have this much pain or so many frustrations? Now I did not have a choice or time to think about why I became a nurse or not. I had to adapt to whatever happened. The fact that the United States at that time had a shortage of nurses was an advantage for me, allowing me to come to America, but it was not easy at all. I was constantly full of fear and stress. I felt so alone. Even more, the hospital didn't know my capabilities when they hired me. There was no test or orientation for English ability at all. I, myself, had to discover what needed to be done and how to do it. I had no time to sleep, like when I was skipped to ninth grade from the sixth in the past. Now I was 33 years old with a family, and it had been a decade since I'd graduated nursing school. With poor reading skills in English, I had to study English and work all day with no sleep. Through all this, working and studying, Insok had to assist me with a ride to and from work, regardless of his workday, and then there were house chores when I got home. Understandably, Insok and I barely slept. For me, the longest I ever slept was four hours. Hardly sleeping and under immense pressure, I became extremely exhausted and stressed as well as confused. Again, I blamed becoming a nurse, and although I was in a paradise country, in the United States, it seemed to me I was wandering a thorny field with no way out. At that time, I felt that having a dream for a better life for me was a complete mistake.

One day, my older daughter told me that she really liked living in the United States because she was able to eat bananas as much as she wanted unlike in South Korea, where they were extremely expensive. By her expression, I sensed that she loved her kindergarten teacher who loved her black hair, although my daughter did not speak English well. My daughter made some friends in the class, and she felt that she was welcomed by them. But she said that she missed her younger sister in Korea as much as I did. In the meantime, I felt that Americans were so friendly, kind, and compassionate, smiling at me as I was passing by and working in broken English. They did not discriminate against me for not speaking well or for being from North Korea. They didn't even care where I was from. Rather, whenever I spoke to patients with my broken English, they tried to understand and help me, explaining to me that learning English is not easy. Even native speakers of English sometimes encountered difficulty. They tried to teach me words and accents with encouragement and said, "You will do OK one day." Also, when I gave instructions to the patients, they listened to me carefully, without frowning, and sincerely respected me because I was a nurse. They tried to comfort me with a smile. I could not forget their encouragement inside of me. Then I said to myself, "This is why Americans were blessed and models for the people." I was developing my voice and would finally be able to express my feelings and emotions; the desire to share all I felt was bigger than the mountains.

I deeply appreciated their compassion, comfort, and attitude, which I felt I did not deserve. In fact, their support taught me and encouraged me to work harder and improve my English as fast as I could. Feeling renewed, I understood why other people wanted to come to America. In the grocery store, I saw how they had fixed prices and displayed the products in an organized way, reminding me of when I was in the PX in Vietnam. Regardless of social rank, no matter how much money I or anyone had, everyone could buy and eat the same things and purchase whatever they needed. This had not been the case in Korea—certain foods were only affordable by wealthier people. But in America, former president Richard Nixon drank the same milk as I did. As someone whose life was so negatively impacted by communism as well as class, I started to question the true meaning of equality, which is foundational to democracy. Never had I considered this. Another thing that impressed me was that no houses seemed to have fences to keep out thieves. Through a big glass window, I remember seeing a whole family eating dinner together in their dining room, under a chandelier. It looked like my dream when I saw it. This observation comforted me and gave me a glimmer of hope and high energy. I said to myself, "When I am ready to bring my baby here, I will have the exact same life."

I promised myself that I would break my frustration to obtain happiness, comfort, and a better life. Reflecting on the thought that I had about making a mistake in coming to the United States, I wondered if I still had the same thoughts that I had previously. Surprisingly, the answer was no. It was different than the feelings that I had at work with the staff at the hospital. I began to discover that the relationships between physicians and nurses were not the same as what I used to see in Korea. I was elated to see the positive perspective on nursing in America. In fact, it was unbelievable. One time, when a patient had a mess on his face, this doctor picked up a towel from the rack to clean the mess rather than asking a nurse to do it. Through this, I felt that there was no sense of class between physicians and nurses when it came to caring for patients. I also observed that physicians and nurses shared charting in the patient's chart; there was not a divided section for physician's only with which I was familiar. I felt that their approach indicated equality for patient care. At the nurse's station, the chair was not reserved for physicians but available to everyone on a first-come-first-served basis. Among the nurses, everyone, from head nurses to staff nurses, was treated the same. The salary of a nurse was enough to support a family with one child as well. While observing these revelations, my agonies and anguish were less bothersome. Seeing this, I could understand why people called America paradise.

But soon enough, I encountered another issue: I received a notice from the hospital that said they were concerned about my proficiency in English, which meant I was not able to become a charge nurse. It looked as though misfortune was always following me. My mind was darker than ever. Even though I understood my imperfect English capability, I could not accept this notice because I knew that I could not learn English overnight. I was absolutely horrified by this situation. My strength and desire all dried out from this notification because I couldn't imagine how long I needed to take time for studying. I was simply desperately overwhelmed, psychologically and physically. I was exhausted, and any newfound hope dissipated. I was struggling to overcome the language barrier and lacked clinical experience. But now I had no solution despite digging deeper for more energy and strength. I wanted to work continuously to learn and improve my life, but I totally lost my passion and desire, feeling numbness. In addition, my last dream was to bring my baby to America under better living conditions. My world was darker than night again. But thankfully, there was light. Sue Chen, a Chinese nurse at the hospital who was around my age, shared with me her previous experience with the language barrier. Understanding my situation, Chen offered to help me since we were on the same shift on the unit. She asked the hospital to schedule both of us during the same shifts because of my English problems. With her help, I perked up and worked diligently with no complaints; I had great appreciation for her and the hospital. After a while, I passed the nursing state board examination to become an RN in the United States. The hospital was pleased that I had finally made it.

Then I requested to be transferred to the Home Visiting Nurse Association in Washington, D.C. This turned out to be an unforgettable experience and a significant memory in my life. I ended up learning about being a home visiting nurse from a coworker, a former nun, who had switched to home visitation. She thought it would be a better fit for me. I was the first immigrant to join the Visiting Nurse Association of Washington, D.C., since it was formed 75 years earlier, in 1900. Not yet realizing how difficult being a home visiting nurse would be, I felt my spirit of hope was higher than ever because I had previous experience working as a public health nurse in South Korea. I felt that this was the one nursing job that I could accomplish to make my dreams come true as a nurse. Also, I thought that this opportunity would teach me about American public health nursing, and I would learn the difference between public health nursing in the United States and South Korea. At the hospital where I had been working, I had not yet felt as though I were achieving the American dream, but transferring to home visitation nursing finally made me feel like my dreams were coming true. All the agonies and frustration from the language barrier and missing my baby seemed to weigh less.

Finally, at this time, my baby and my mother-in-law arrived safely and joined us. With good care from Young Kyu, my baby had grown tall and healthy, and she was beautiful and spoke Korean well. When I'd left her behind, she could only crawl. Now she walked and danced as a girl. She was totally different, and I was indescribably happy. I'd missed her so much, day and night. The missing never left me. But she was now in front of me once again and it almost felt like I was in a dream. I fully paid respect to Young Kyu for caring for my daughter like when I was in Vietnam. At first, my baby called me her aunt, not recognizing me as her mother. She was used to not seeing me or using the word "mom" while she was in South Korea. That made me sad—I didn't respond to "aunt" but just cried. My daughter thinking of me as

V—Seeking the American Dream

her aunt and not her mother indicated that so much time had passed. She was just shy of four years old, too young to warrant explaining why I'd left her with Young Kyu, whom my daughter considered to be her mother. She couldn't sleep at night without my mother-in-law nearby. It took almost two years for my daughter to understand that I was her mother, and when she realized this, it made the sacrifices, moving to the United States and establishing a safe life for her here, all worth it. Since Vietnam, the sadness, agony, suffering, and missing my daughter seemed permanent, but carrying on, seeing her again, showed it was never in vain.

In this moment, I looked back to see how I had managed to live with all the pain, frustrations, and sufferings, but I had enough help to deal with these horrible situations. I now had reached the point where I could see that my lovely, healthy daughter was living safely with my mother-in-law. I began to acknowledge that I'd only ever focused on the difficult aspects of my life, not seeing the good side because I selfishly needed to survive. I had just focused on only these difficult problems. But now I was able to see things differently in appreciation, and I realized that life was not under my control. There was something that I couldn't answer for the mystery and eternity in the space. Finally, I admitted that God must be there with me all along with no touch, no sound, and no visibility, which I'd never believed before because of all that had happened. Until then, somehow, I recognized that God would always be there to protect me.

I had never felt that because real life was too harsh and different than what had been preached to me when I was young. But God had, in fact, helped me because I felt that His help was "mercy and love and grace." Later I found out that I was blind, dull, and deaf to not recognize Him at all. Realizing God's love, grace, and mercy, I had a new view and perspective on the world from dark to light which I simply initially resisted to admit due to all the grievous hardships through three wars, crossing the DMZ. I couldn't and hadn't believed in God, ignoring my father's heritage. When I investigated my past at this point, I always had some sort of help, but I didn't recognize what it was. I confessed that I did not have the power to control or remain resilient through everything that was happening. I admitted that I was wrong about God. I didn't know about myself, how I'd often been weak and ignorant, but thankfully, my desire or motivation to learn never stopped except nursing. With God, I began to believe there was a new world, where my eyes were opened and I was enlightened so that I was able to discover what I didn't know and what I had to know about my life and my daughter, who was so close to her grandmother, my mother-in-law. (She ended up writing her college admission essay about Young Kyu.) I learned how good God was and is for ultimately leading me to my dream life. I felt less fear, anxiety, and agonies because I depended on my belief in God. In the past, I tended to be negative, envying other people who had had an easier life. I blamed myself that I should have understood better the story of Job in the Old Testament, focusing on chapter 42, verse 1–6: "Job answered the Lord: I know that you can do all things and that no purpose is beyond you. You ask: who is this obscuring counsel yet lacking knowledge? But I have spoken of things which I have not understood, things too wonderful for me to know. Listen, and let me speak. You said: I shall put questions to you, and you must answer. I knew of you then only by report, but now I see you with my own eyes. Therefore I yield, repenting in dust and ashes."

Now I appreciated that I had been through the difficulties; they taught me about life. I found new values, and my entire perspective changed from negative to positive—my mind was opened. In other words, I let go of the anger in my heart and unchained myself from old cultural frames.

I had to learn how to drive a car for my job as a home visiting nurse. So my husband taught me how to drive our car. I learned about the city plan of Washington, D.C., which was done in the most scientific way in the world. Capitol Hill was the center of Washington, D.C., where it was the main landmark. Odd and even numbers were used to order addresses and provide directions, unlike in Korea, where this numbering was not used. Also, the street names were organized in alphabetical order, using the names of famous people (Abraham for "A") and fruits (apple for "A"), and the pattern went in all cardinal directions. I was amazed to learn it. As a newcomer, I did not have many problems finding the houses and making the four or five visits daily. Because I knew the layout, I did not struggle, even though my English was still not strong. I once even helped a fellow nurse, who was born and raised

V—Seeking the American Dream

in America, with directions in D.C. because she never knew the city plan. She said jokingly, "We are always learning until we die."

While visiting the homes of Medicaid beneficiaries in northern D.C., I was quickly shocked by some observations and unexpected situations, where the families were so poor that they had no lights and their windows were broken. They did not have air conditioners. When visiting patients, I always had to wash my hands in the bathroom or kitchen, and both rooms always revealed how unfortunately many of these people lived. Some families were poorer than my own when we were living in South Korea. I was shocked and surprised about how the people lived, but they respected me because I was a nurse, and even though I could not speak English that well, they spoke to me in English with kindness, warmth, and sincerity. I reflected on how the Americans helped us during the Korean War. Then I wondered how America helped us even when people lived at home in this condition. It was surprising for me to see such poverty. I always knew that America was known as a place of paradise on earth, but the scenes that I saw were very much different and opposite from what I'd heard. It was not as simple as I'd hoped. However, it was a useful opportunity, and I wondered about the many possible reasons and meanings behind this hidden reality. I wished to write these observations in English, but it was impossible due to my English skills. But I learned that the most important thing was how to practice, as the Bible says, to "love your neighbor as yourself" (Matthew 22:39). I felt that this learning was more than gold. This helped me to understand the relationships between America and Korea during wartime. I recalled all the help by the Americans from my old memories from the tent life after crossing the DMZ and my time during the wars.

Another significant impression was that almost every house had a picture of Jesus, Abraham Lincoln, and Martin Luther King, Jr., in varying sizes. One house had an entire wall covered in pictures of Jesus. I was taken aback; I was Christian, but wherever I moved, I felt Jesus watching me; in fact, I disliked it. Since having that experience, I began to question how to believe in Jesus. Further, I opened my eyes, learning of various ways of believing or having religion. It was a unique experience. Still, seeing the picture of Jesus remains in my memory nonstop.

From North Korea to America Through Three Wars

Occasionally, I met veterans from the Korean War who remembered the places where they had been stationed. Also, kimchi and Korean barbecue were the most unforgettable things in their memories. Some even asked if I would make kimchi, which they loved after trying despite not liking the smell. The veterans also remembered Korean women as being beautiful and sweet but that Korea was extremely cold in the winter. The veterans always treated me with kindness; they were happy to see me because they recalled their old memories. They wanted to go back to Korea to see how it had changed, but they could not afford it. Many of the veterans were poor, and I wondered why, but I was not fluent enough in English to ask any further questions.

Through these home visits, I had learned many things like the differences between government-run Medicaid and Medicare benefits in the U.S. healthcare system. In South Korea, when you were not feeling well, you saw a private doctor in the neighborhood, whereas in the United States, you made an appointment or could go to the emergency room. I also learned about the role of visiting nurses, which did not exist back home. There was no system of home visiting nurses like with U.S. healthcare, and nursing was so much more different in the States than in Korea. It was complicated for me to understand all those rules and policies in English, but I had to work with it, sensing that I was gaining a new concept of nursing. It was a huge challenge to learn those things as much as at the hospital, requiring more English writing skills and being independent during home visiting.

In 1975, much to my surprise, First Lady Betty Ford invited the Visiting Nurses Association of Washington, D.C., to the White House to celebrate the organization's 75th anniversary. As a nurse, I was shocked that I was invited to the White House, especially for me, who'd grown up in Korea, where nurses were seen as maids. When Mrs. Ford cut the association's birthday cake, I was on the South Lawn of the White House. All of us visiting nurses were treated as special guests and were free to explore the first and second floors of the White House except for Mrs. Ford's bedroom and private areas. Thanks to former first lady Jacqueline Kennedy, each room was a different color, which indicated the art, music, and guests. It was a special moment that opened my eyes. I saw all the first lady portraits and was

V—Seeking the American Dream

impressed by Jacqueline Kennedy's portrait because it was not a typical classical painting. It was very modern for the time. I also saw the china collection from former first lady Eleanor Roosevelt on display. I adopted that idea for my personal life as well and put together my own china cabinet. At one point, I was satisfied that I was able to work in Washington, D.C., without needing to take my examination to come to the United States, which would've been impossible for me to pass. I loved learning American history and culture and Americans' way of life, including visiting the White House for this special occasion. The meaning of this visit was abundance to me when I look back at my life. Among the many nurses on that day, I might be the only one who felt such an impact.

This visit to the White House made me think deeply and enjoy more living in the United States. I had reflected on what my American dream was. In my dream, I never had a dream about buying a big house or living a luxurious lifestyle that focused on materialism. Rather, I

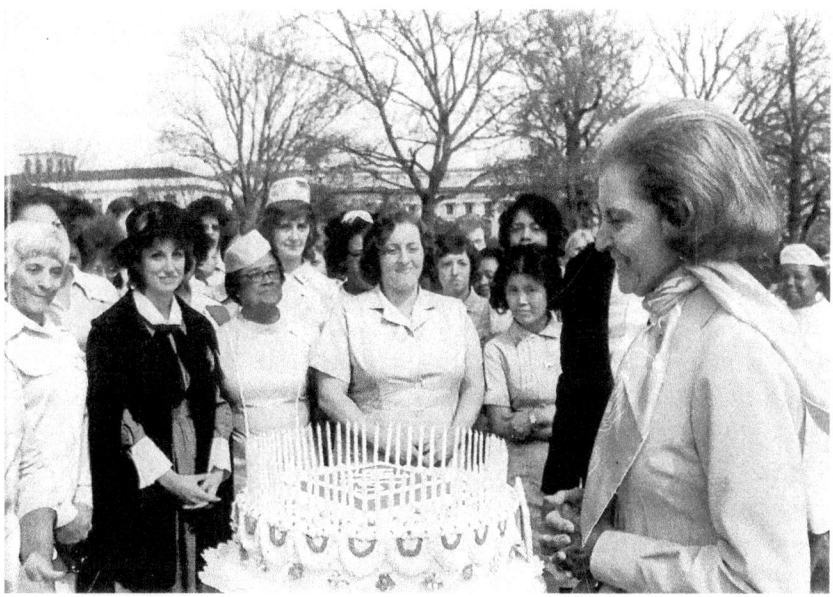

First Lady Betty Ford shares a cake with members of the Washington, D.C., Visiting Nurses Association at the White House, 1975. Sung Yoo is fifth from left in the row of nurses. Official White House photograph by Karl Schumacher.

wanted to learn English and study whatever I wanted to learn about unknown things in the world because I hadn't had any choice what I want to study. Now I was beginning to see a different world by learning English and even getting an invitation to visit the White House as a nurse. This would not have happened in Korea. It was a good chance to observe the cultural differences of the West and East. In the White House because of the anniversary of the Home Visiting Nurse Association, I imagined that as a home visiting nurse in Korea, I wouldn't ever be invited to the Blue House, the residence of the president of South Korea. The treatment of nurses was just not the same in the two countries. This treatment could be added to my American dream.

But the feelings of happiness did not last long. My conversational English had improved immensely with staff and patients. Also, I was building good relationships with the patients and coworkers, but writing reports and recording charts still proved difficult. I was able to do more because I had experience at the hospital, but I was unable to keep stride with other home visiting nurses because of the reports. It was much harder than I expected, especially the written reports, which were so important for Medicaid and Medicare, as they were government documents. So I usually brought work home and had no time to spend with family because I had to finish reports. It was the writing that made me put in the extra hours every day. At the hospital, I needed to write up reports on the patients' physical conditions and what I did and observed at that time. But at the home visit, I needed to write comprehensive assessments of large scope, such as the family structure, financial conditions, and physical condition in which they lived, which was quite different than the hospital. This was difficult for me since I was not familiar with the system. I discovered myself where I lacked knowledge. I needed to have analytical skills as well as evaluation skills about the whole situation. Being a home visiting nurse, I needed to be independent and gain a greater understanding of the complex living situations of those I visited, which was quite different than what hospital nurses had to know. I asked other nurses who had no English problems, but they had the same complaints, understanding how hard it could be. I kept trying to follow up and make time for the reports, but I realized that my ability prevented me from continuing this line of work. I learned that writing English was different than

V—Seeking the American Dream

speaking English. My speaking level was higher than my reading or writing level. It was a big moment again to learn what the differences were between speaking, reading, and writing English. I discovered by myself that I had to jump to a much higher level for reading and writing. Then I recognized that my foundation was weak. It was hard and difficult for me to confront because it was impossible to improve in writing English overnight, and it absolutely terrified me. I began to lose weight due to increased stress. Finally, I decided to resign after one year.

Simultaneously, my mother-in-law, who had been helping me a lot around the house, had to go back to Korea after staying with us for two years. Her help had allowed me to work as a home visiting nurse. It was a great experience being a home visiting nurse in Washington, D.C., because I had a chance to learn about the city plan and structure as well as how the veterans of the Korean War had lived. I never had an idea of how the American soldiers were in their native place before and after war. In addition, I learned how hard writing in English was for a beginner like me with a poor foundation. So I was able to focus on writing and reading for my English improvement. I was grateful for lessons for English study. I wanted to share these experiences with anybody who wanted to learn and to teach English.

Then, by this time, we had to move to Princeton, New Jersey, for my husband's business in August 1976, America's bicentennial birthday. When I moved to Princeton, I saw American flags displayed all over downtown, at Nassau Hall, and the Dinky station. Soon after we moved, I decided to study English harder and attended Mercer County Community College (MCCC) only to study the language. With my experience from being a home visiting nurse, I felt that learning to write in English was more important than before. Also, I remembered an older Czechoslovakian woman at the hospital in Washington, D.C., who could barely speak English, even though she had lived in the United States for 15 years. She was unable to ask me in English for a pair of scissors, and I did not want to be like her having struggles for a simple thing. I became set on improving my English. It took almost 25 minutes driving through cornfields to get to school. It was my time to be happy to go to school. I was greatly happy to learn English in the classroom from an American teacher.

From North Korea to America Through Three Wars

Often, I felt that my dream came true like other people said. My time studying in America was unlike studying nursing in Korea. I received compliments from some students about my attitude toward learning, and they admired that I was older, which was totally opposite from my past in nursing class, when I felt shame for being the oldest in the class. In fact, at MCCC, I was praised for being an older student, which was a huge encouragement. It was another cultural difference that made me happy; I was proud to be the oldest student. I never expected it. My goal was to read the *New York Times* so I could share the news with my children in English. Up to this point, I could only read the big titles, not the stories or editorials.

Once in the class, the professor offered to tutor me for free in English because he said that he had never seen a student like me who wanted to study so hard. I read European literature, which was the first time in my life I encountered the *Iliad* by Homer, *War and Peace* by Leo Nikolayevich Tolstoy, and *Oliver Twist* by Charles Dickens. I still remember reading when Achilles killed Hector, the prince of Troy, and Hector's father, King Priam, went to retrieve his son's body. Although they were enemies, Achilles and Priam embraced each other and cried together over their losses. I learned from here through literature from antiquity what humanity meant, something to which I had never paid attention. I was moved and touched deeply. This was a new useful learning. There was no enemy in front of death, just human life. Although these well-known authors were all dead, they brought me into a new world. I discovered that I did not know how much I did not know. I was in a narrow and small world as a human being. I regretted that I did not study hard enough to know how this literature helped to open my eyes to see the world. I said to myself that literature is a lens through which we can see the lives in the world. Truly, I did not know how important literature was. At this time, for the first time in my life, I related the meaning of literature to nursing care. Learning this value of literature incited in me my eagerness which could boost the rich life inside of me. The minute I felt this feeling, I was so happy, like the whole world was mine. The sky looked bluer, teaching me that the world was not what I had seen, which was small. It was larger and higher and wider. That experience had never happened to me until now. I never knew about literature being powerful and shining like the stars.

V—Seeking the American Dream

In the meantime, being home to study English, I was pregnant with a son. My husband was especially excited to have a son because he felt that his last name would be carried on after him by the first son of his family in the Korean tradition. Of course, we were all happy about my pregnancy. I felt that I was too old to have a baby, but it happened. Even church members were so happy, like he was their own child. Especially the minister felt this baby was born by God's blessing in our church. I hadn't had a chance to raise my own child till this time. The whole family was full of joy with a new healthy baby, named Hans. Furthermore, when I thought that I might have a chance to raise a child on my own, I wanted to enjoy every moment because previously, I did not have time to bathe a newborn and play with two daughters. Everywhere in our house was full of smiles and new life.

Then, again, I had a question about what I should do after having a son. I wanted to continue to work for my own self-development. If my English continued to improve, I thought I might study sociology or philosophy, disciplines in which I had to read many books, but I felt that my English was not strong enough yet. When Hans became one year old, I started to work as a part-time staff nurse at Merwick, a long-term care facility at Princeton Medical Center because nursing was my major subject still. I needed to prepare for my future in the United States. When I went to have an interview at Merwick, the residents all looked like big white rabbits because their hair was all white, and they were motionless, shrunken, and bent to the front, some sleeping in wheelchairs. It was depressing and unpleasant, but I reminded myself that I had to work here because it was convenient. It was not far from my home, and I worked only the day shift. Additionally, I was curious about how the American elderly were treated in Western culture. I thought it might be a good chance to compare Eastern and Western approaches to elder care. Traditionally, in the East, elder care should be done at home by the family, unlike in the West. By looking, the working conditions were not pleasant because it was smelly and dark in the room, and everybody moved slowly. The residents were not very animated. Simply, it was not at all attractive to me, but I felt that I would end up like these residents—it was only a matter of time. After a visit to Merwick, I thought deeply about end-of-life issues. Regardless of whether we lived in Eastern or Western cultures, all have to face eventual death at home or in a facility like Merwick. In the modern world, there are higher chances of dying in facilities like Merwick.

Eventually, I enrolled in a master's course in gerontological nursing education at Villanova University. The first class was about nursing theory, which I had never heard of or could understand the concepts at first. However, I felt marvelous and wonderful to be in this class even though it was hard to comprehend the whole theory. I was surprised that nursing has a theory like other professions, and it fascinated me. At least I understood that nursing theory allowed for the development of a body of knowledge regarding the concepts and backbone of the practice which I had so abhorred. I was amazed to hear that nursing could be a profession, which made me so proud for enrolling at Ewha Womans University in Seoul. My eagerness to learn nursing theory had increased and encouraged me to study more about nursing. I was so glad that I was learning the theory as others. All nursing theorists were new, unlike old traditional theories like in philosophy, psychology, and religion. With the increased desire, I began to ask what nursing was, which was the basic question and knowledge of nursing. I regretted that I had not known these questions at the beginning in nursing school. By questioning, I was awakened to how careless and ignorant I had been about nursing.

With this awakening, I asked myself what I knew about nursing. I felt desolate as a nurse. Being aware of that, I felt that I was blind. Ironically, being blind, I was able to see clearly about myself, who was too dull, senseless, close minded, and simple. I was in deep speculation and meditation about myself, how and why I had been so prejudiced against nursing and the view that it was an inferior occupation.

Now I wanted to be a nurse until the end of my life. I had to be different than before. I began to search for a way of being changed, a new nurse with an old heart. I reviewed life from my childhood on. I was known well in town among villagers and friends, but while growing up and through marriage, I had rough times, experiencing rejection and discrimination with many conflicting ideas that could not be answered and explained. It was too early for me to face all of that. Then, rather than accept the frustrations, I hurt even more and tried to escape from the struggles, which were rooted in social and cultural aspects, such as class. I became so sensitive to that concept and wanted to avoid being a nurse who usually had a low reputation in Korean society. I never thought of giving care to sick people belonging to a lower class. Rather, I wanted to be higher class like when I was a child in my hometown. I believed that if I became a nurse for my entire life, I would always be seen as a lower class person than what I wanted to be. For this reason, I did not want to be a nurse. But now I realized how wrong I was for having those concepts. I did not want to be that kind of old nurse, but I wanted to be a new nurse who had changed and was transformed. Surprisingly, through this review of my young life, I discovered that I had been deeply attached to Confucianism naturally. I did not want to be in it, but I was there, too.

Realizing my prejudice toward nursing, I like to quote the Bible: "I knew you then only by report, but now I see you with my own eyes. Therefore, I yield repenting in dust and ashes" (Job 42:6). With this new learning, I felt that Merwick was not the same as it once was. I treated this place as a philosophy center, not a smelly, long-term care facility. I realized that the impression that I'd had of the residents at the beginning as old rabbits was totally wrong. In addition, the residents appealed as human lives, carriers of truth in my senses. Like in literature, the facility demonstrated humanity, how life endured. Learning nursing theories, I began to recognize that nursing was all about life and death, which I should've known earlier and practiced with more sincerity and understanding. At this point, I recalled and admired Florence Nightingale, who had developed nursing theory, as well as the nursing theorists who followed her. I wanted to know more about her for my own good. Then I hoped to find out what was different between her and me or what could be the same.

VI

Florence Nightingale[1]

On August 15, 1910, two days after Florence Nightingale died, the *New York Times* published, "The chorus of praise which reached her ears as she sat in her invalid's chair at the completion of threescore years and ten was such as few women have enjoyed in the history of the world."[2] Surely, there have been few people who inspired so many. I was surprised when I read this century-old statement about Nightingale, who I only knew as "the Lady with the Lamp." Even though I was a nurse, I knew nothing about Nightingale, nor did I have any interest in learning about her life. But I came to find out that she essentially created the art of professional nursing—nowadays called modern nursing—and changed the view of nursing from a lowly and often discredited occupation. Nightingale also reframed nursing to make sure all people, including those less fortunate and sick, received care for their well-being, which is something I wish I'd learned much earlier.[3] The more I studied her work, the more I discovered that my nursing knowledge was abysmal and that I lacked any insight into nursing as a nurse.

    I felt ashamed and distressed as I was awakened to my own selfishness and narrow-mindedness. For me, I'd already had countless benevolences as a nurse during the Vietnam War and in the United States. At this moment, I was shocked by how foolish I'd been. I recalled how I behaved when Sung Kul suggested that I apply to nursing school. While being a nurse, I had a better life, as my brother promised. However, I was still completely blind to what nursing was all about. My eyes were closed in the nursing world, but thankfully an epic transformation occurred from a negative way of thinking about nursing to a more positive view. Right after this change, I was not the

VI—Florence Nightingale

same nurse as I once was. I was a beginner in nursing—a new nurse with an old heart. I wished I had a chance to fix how selfish and disgraceful I'd been. One benefit for a new beginner was that I had more desire to study nursing, repenting how I felt toward nursing in the past. After a long time of holding resentment, I realized Sung Kul was right. With this epiphany, I sincerely thanked my brother and told him I appreciated his guidance from the bottom of my heart.

When I read about the life story of Nightingale, I realized that there were some commonalities and differences between us, which impressed and surprised me. For her in the 19th century and me growing up in Korea, nursing was regarded as a lackluster profession, and nurses were seen as doctors' helpers, barely above a housemaid. From there, however, we set off in different directions in nursing. While I still maintained a negative perception of nursing and only showed up to work to receive a paycheck, Nightingale took on the establishment to incite change as a nurse. With a determined mind, she wanted to create the discipline of what would become modern professional nursing. She made it her life's work, even not marrying because of it.

Nightingale insisted that nursing education should develop both intellect and character and include a solid background in the sciences to enable nurses to understand the theory behind their care. When I learned about her opinion of care on nursing, I respected and admired her approach to nursing.[4] It was completely opposite from the way I had approached nursing. She saw nursing as a very noble profession, while I was still disparaging it and seeking to avoid it. The difference was day and night. However, I was enlightened by her and began to ask questions about the occupation. Up until this moment, I'd never thought of nursing like she had; I had much regret that I did not pay any attention to nursing theory while living in Korea and Vietnam. Then she added that without nursing theory, nursing cannot be a profession. This statement was a revolution in the nursing world, especially for me. I'd only ever obeyed the doctor's order and never considered the definition of care in nursing or even thought to question what it all might mean. Before I understood the concept of "care" through nursing theory, I did not know how important it was for the well-being of people, rich or poor, man or woman, old or young. Care represented usually helping sick people, which is close to nursing. But now, influenced by Nightingale, my attitude toward caring or nursing was changed, and I began to have a new understanding of nursing as a caring profession. It should come from studying philosophy, science, religion, literature, and sociology, all of which are required to determine true nursing. Understanding this notion, I became an entirely different nurse.

From all this new concept of nursing, I was more appreciative of being a nurse. Naturally, I paid more respect to Nightingale for enlightening me. I agreed with her idea that nurses need to study the humanities for an increased understanding of human lives. Thinking of my own experience, before I even studied Nightingale, I had the same thought about the humanities. That made me so happy. When I had studied European literature at the MCCC in New Jersey, these insights from the literature were fresh and new to me. I wish that I had more chances to teach the new nurses about this necessity of literature. After all, I was so glad that I had one thing in common with Florence Nightingale despite our different backgrounds and experiences.

Another point was Nightingale's statement that a nurse should never stop learning, which I also believed even before I studied her. From my own experiences, I sensed that nursing has been deeply related to life and death. But the meaning of nursing was not as well defined as was the case with other professions. At least I had some commonality with Nightingale, which encouraged me. Actually, I hoped that I might have another chance to teach this necessity to the future nurses, focusing on literature. I hope this book will inspire future nurses to never stop learning, including reading humanities literature. I do really wish that.

Then I began to wonder how Nightingale had such advanced ideas in nursing and brilliant writing skills for her time. She wrote about 45 books including *Notes on Nursing: What Is Nursing and What It Is Not*, focused on professional nursing and issues concerning sanitation in both army and civilian hospitals, hygiene, and statistics.[5] At that time, she didn't even attend school at all because she was female. Not only that, before she went to the Crimean War (1854–1856), at the age of 30 she began to write her book *Suggestions for Thought* and finished it after she returned home in 1860; it consists of three volumes—two volumes on philosophy and one on religion. This book is highly

VI—Florence Nightingale

intellectual, philosophical, and religious and was intended for the artisans of England, telling them to believe in God in their lives. This book was read and commented on by two famous men, John Stuart Mill and Benjamin Jowett. The criticism was different between them: Mill said it was ready to be published, whereas Jowett said it needed revisions. But Jowett wished to publish it more than Mill did. Jowett met Nightingale, and their relationship grew until the end of his life. Although they never married, he wished Nightingale could be by his side when he passed away. The book was not published in her lifetime, but it stands as a remarkable work. No one could read it without being impressed by her writing skills, powerful mind, and spirituality.[6]

On May 12, 1820, Nightingale was born to English parents while on a trip to Florence, Italy. Growing up in England, she never wanted to marry, although her mother insisted on it. Because she had no interest in marriage, unlike her sister Penelope, Nightingale had a bad relationship with her mother. On the other hand, her father was very open minded and understood her wants in her life. Nightingale learned from her father, a Cambridge graduate, who supported her and taught her philosophy, statistics, literature, the Bible, and multiple languages including Latin. I was inspired by the way she learned from her father, as it reminded me of how my father was like Nightingale's. My father had almost the same strength, desire, and motivation to learn and teach his children without having gone to school himself.[7]

My father's teaching methods were so strict. He believed that human beings were different from animals because of education. He taught us how to speak and greet the elderly. When any child did not follow in his way, we used to get hit by a hard stick on the palm or calves. Then he explained why we got hit, and he kept a careful record of these punishments which he showed us. No one else in our hometown compared with his desire for education. In particular, he emphasized that we must not use vulgar words. If we did, then it was another hit.

Thankfully, my father was able to give me the heritage that I could carry on until now although I was slow and dull. Nightingale was able to keep going in nursing with her father's support and his understanding because they had a close relationship. My father died when I was still young, so our relationship never had the chance to become like theirs. But his spirit and strength remained in me. Even though Nightingale's mother and Penelope strongly advised her to marry, Nightingale kept studying and writing. Instead, she was looking for work that would allow her to be independent in her life. Unhappy with her family except for her father, she wanted to help people, doing God's work. From July through October 1851, Nightingale went to Kaiserswerth, a hospital near Düsseldorf in Germany that trained volunteer nurses. She was impressed by the hospital, feeling that it was very different than home. She worked not with a program but with her heart, something I should've done but never did. There, Nightingale found her calling and was able to gain valuable experience helping others, learning the importance of morals. She felt that while she was there, her world was filled with joy and interest, and she strengthened her body and mind. Those three months she spent at Kaiserswerth were a turning point in her career, but they were not as effective as she'd hoped. She went on to serve additional apprenticeships in nursing in Paris hospitals, where she diligently collected data of hospital organizations and nursing arrangements, but she never had formal nursing education or obtained a degree like me. She had different opportunities to give care to her father, her aunt Evans, and her grandmother before their deaths. Later, she continued to serve her apprenticeship in Paris, and she became a charge nurse at an institution on Harley Street in London. But the news from the *Times* about the Crimean War was about to change her future.[8]

The *Times* reported on the overall poor medical situation and preparation of the British army during the Crimean War. Not only was there a lack of surgeons but also medical supplies and "dressers," or nurses. The *Times* said that the French were superior to the British when it came to medical care, and the French had help from devoted women like nurses, such as the Sisters of Charity. The newspaper asked why the British lacked such care. Nightingale was inspired to help after reading the news on the poor conditions.[9]

At this time, British secretary at war Sidney Herbert, who was "deeply interested … in the care of the sick" but "had nothing to do with war," had "pondered long over the problems of nursing, both in military hospitals and in civil life." Since he heard that the French government had sent out the Sisters of Charity, he thought England

VI—Florence Nightingale

should do something similar. With input from his wife, Herbert considered Nightingale, who had long been prepared for such work. Herbert, his wife, and Nightingale collaborated to rally nurses to be sent to Crimea to improve medical conditions for soldiers.[10]

On October 21, 1854, Nightingale left London for Crimea with 38 nurses to serve the sick and suffering, hoping greatly to extend the scope of her work. On November 4, she arrived safely at Scutari, where some of the military officers welcomed her, while the others resented her and her staff. She kept calm and composed, showing herself to be efficient and helpful, applying an expert's touch among the doctors. On the day of Nightingale's arrival, the wounded were pouring in fast. All staff worked wonderfully, being useful and efficient during the worst surgical cases. Their reputation was raised, and nothing critical could be said of their work. Nightingale reported to the commander of the forces about their poor working conditions, including torn-off roofs, broken windows, no water, backed-up sewer lines, pests, and air with no ventilation, all of which resulted in gross neglect of the sick and wounded and even sicker patients.[11]

The hospital lacked basic comforts and necessities such as bed linens, utensils, blankets, sheets, and surgical and medical supplies. At that time, dysentery, cholera, and typhus were rampant. Despite their kindness, clever judgment, and intelligence, every nurse's work was impossible during this difficult mission. Nightingale began to work in the Barrack Hospital in three ways: applying an expert's touch, assuming bold responsibilities, and writing the authorities at home to improve these conditions.[12]

According to Sir Edward Cook in *The Life of Florence Nightingale Vol. 1 (1820–1861)*, Nightingale considered the soldiers to be her children, and the wounded men said with tears, "She thinks of us" and "I only wish I could go and fight for her again." Cook continued, explaining that those to whom she wrote letters said, "Each man of us ought to have a copy from Nightingale which we will keep till our dying day." Queen Victoria even sent a message, demonstrating substantial proof of Her Majesty's interest. She wrote, "Miss Nightingale was made the intermediary between the throne and the soldiers." Nightingale's popularity was not limited to the letters from soldiers in Crimea and their homes. She was called by old soldiers "the Lady with the Lamp."[13]

From North Korea to America Through Three Wars

When Nightingale returned home, the government had offered her a British man-of-war ship for the voyage home, but she declined, avoiding a public celebration because she had carefully withheld information on her time schedules from her family. She was humble. She arrived home on August 7, 1856, walking up from the little country station, "a little tinkle of the small church bell" in the distance.[14]

Immediately, Nightingale set to work upon her return. Many were surprised that she did not take enough rest after returning. She realized that no one knew how soldiers were treated, while the people at home fed their own children and dressed them in silk and velvet. The poor sanitary conditions on the battlefield resulted in many soldiers dying during the dreadful winters. Nightingale could not forget their graves. She began to tabulate the causes of their deaths. She summarized and analyzed the figures during her residence in the Crimean hospitals, reviewing the deaths of 4,600 soldiers. Her personal observations and statistical inquiries, "the most complete experiment ever conducted on army hygiene," proved that the terrible rate of mortality could be reduced. She was awakened to the neglect, feeling deep pity for the victims of preventable disease. She continued to examine hospital statistics in London and the "complete lack of scientific coordination." After the war, Nightingale reported to the Royal Commission to describe the state of the Barrack Hospital. The senior chaplain had the sense to recognize Nightingale as an admirable person and a perfect lady. She did many things herself but gave recognition to others for their assistance. I was so impressed by her attitude, mindset, and achievements because I'd never imagined that a nurse could accomplish such feats. Nightingale widened my own scope of what nursing could be; it was very much bigger and deeper than just following a doctor's orders.[15]

Nightingale was one of the most famous people who contributed to the relief of human suffering due to disease in England. She was "the founder of modern nursing," essentially creating "nursing as a trained profession." When I understood her contribution to modern nursing as a trained profession, I was grateful to learn that I had the similar idea through my own practice. It is because I had an experience that giving care to my patients required ongoing education not only in subjects related to nursing but also philosophy, literature,

VI—Florence Nightingale

religion, etc. Nursing requires a holistic point of view for care. I was so moved by her innovative approach to nursing practice even though she had never attended schools to learn any of her nursing skills like I had. I was amazed about her creative approach during her practice in Crimea. She identified the root causes of the number of dead soldiers. At that time, it was hard to distinguish the source of death. Even doctors were clueless. It was difficult to tell whether soldiers were dead because of gunshots or infection. However, she used a statistical tablet that she developed and discovered the importance of sanitary practices which is the core of nursing practice. Through her research, she found how important it is to prevent cross-infection through nursing practice. Her practice and compassion toward wounded soldiers saved their lives.[16]

At the beginning of the Crimean War, her reports were initially treated lightly because she was a female and a nurse during the Victorian era in England. As time went by, the government used her reports to improve sanitary policies for the army and civilians. While I was reading her life story, I was amazed by her works and thoughts on nursing; I had never thought about using statistics in nursing care. It was a huge awakening for me.[17] At first, I'd had no interest in learning nursing theory behind the profession due to my own stereotypes of nursing, and I never wondered whether the theory existed or not. Through the course requirement at Villanova University, I had a chance to learn about it, and I read *Nursing Theories: The Base for Professional Nursing Practice* by Julie B. George. Thankfully, I used this discovery to learn about the nursing theories from Nightingale. The more I studied and the more I read about Nightingale, the more I came to respect and admire her theories. It was a big turning point from being blind to opening my eyes by her works. I wished I had known her much earlier.

Then, learning about Nightingale, my perspective toward the patients and staff at Merwick changed. Now I gave sympathy to a coworker who used to say that if I were married to a rich man, I wouldn't have to work this job. I used to agree with her before. But with my changed values of nursing, I couldn't agree with her anymore. My practice at Merwick was not the same as it once was. I began to have a deeper understanding toward most nursing assistants who always worked harder than any other employees at hospitals or long-term care facilities, having two to three different jobs because they had children. They always lacked much-needed sleep. However, they were not recognized for what they did by staff or patients and their families. They needed the most emotional support by RNs. I tried to help nursing assistants, which RNs often didn't do. One morning, at the busiest time for breakfast, one mildly demented resident had no dentures and couldn't remember where he kept them. His nursing assistant had no idea how she could help him after she searched everywhere possible. Then this resident said that he'd put them in the trash can after dinner, but the trash can was already empty by the morning shift. I empathized with this nursing assistant, who was awfully busy, because she did not want to dig through the dumpster. I was obviously busy, but I spent about 30 minutes that morning rummaging through the trash, but I didn't find the dentures. I was so desperate to find the dentures because of respect for the Patient Rights Law and his inability to eat food. At that moment, his wife came to feed him and brought his dentures with her. I was anxiously telling her about how we'd been unable to find them. She said that she'd taken them home last night, not realizing how diligently we'd tried to find them. If I had not understood nursing, I would've been disappointed by her and upset that I worked that hard without recognition. But I was rather pleased that I could help the nursing assistant, who was very appreciative of me understanding the work. She expressed sincerely to me that she had never had support from an RN in her past. We became so close after this incident.

Another time, there was a severe snowstorm, and a patient's daughter from Baltimore, Maryland, who was close with her father couldn't visit him and stay overnight in Princeton. She called me and explained her fears and concerns regarding her father's care. She said that she missed him and wanted to see him more than before due to the weather. She hoped to be with her father to comfort him. I assured her that he would receive the same care whether she was there or not. Her father would be the same. Then, trusting my words, she decided not to visit her father in the bad weather. Later, to express her appreciation, she bought me a gold bracelet, saying that she was able to

VI—Florence Nightingale

relax and sleep well because she worried about her father that night. Assisting this family could be counted as community nursing care, saving energy and cost, and cutting down on any risk of danger due to bad weather. This simple telephone conversation looked easy, but it was related to the deep meaning of nursing definition concerning the family situation, comforting their concern, something that I previously lacked. Again, Nightingale's *Notes on Nursing* inspired this new insight about nursing. Over the years, I received countless thank-you cards and letters from the families and residents who felt that I was different from others. Whenever I got these recognitions, I thought of Nightingale, how much she had meant to me.

In 2005, I decided to leave Merwick because I received the opportunity to assist Korean nurses at Eastern University. At this point, I wanted to share with the Korean nurses what I'd learned through my own experiences and from Nightingale. I knew about the Korean nurses, who might have almost the same experiences in nursing that I had in Korea. I wanted to show them how my views on nursing had changed and what nursing was truly about. On my final day at Merwick, the whole staff, fellow nurses, janitors, and housekeepers, presented me with a plaque that read, "Never to Be Lost Are the Imprints of People Who Have Changed Our Lives, People Who Have Influenced and Inspired Our Futures, Friends Who Will Forever Remain a Part of Us." Some staff who had the day off, a very precious day for them, attended my farewell party, bringing homemade dishes in crockpots, saying that I should not leave, calling me their queen. When I stepped out of Merwick one final time, a nursing assistant whom I had grown close to came to me, hugged me with tears in her eyes, and said, "Do you have to go? I know you must go." Still, I remember her tears that looked like stars.

Another nursing assistant, Valerie, rushed to me saying that she had decided to go to nursing school although she had two jobs, because she was inspired by me to learn English, to understand and have good relationships with nursing assistants, and to adapt to a different culture. She thought about her circumstances, comparing herself with me, and decided to study nursing. She discovered that her spoken English was much better than mine as well as her English reading skills, which were huge advantages. She wanted to copy my way of building a good relationship with the other nursing assistants. Working with Valerie further encouraged me to teach the Korean nursing students what I had learned from Florence Nightingale, a great inspiration for all nurses.

VII

Mother, Grandmother, Sister, Counselor, Teacher, Nurse

In the fall of 2005, I joined the Eastern University Department of Nursing RN-to-BSN program for South Korean nurses as a director and eventually a lecturer. The program at Eastern University in Pennsylvania was based on Eastern University's mission and philosophy:

"The Students in the BSN Program are given an opportunity for a life of service as a professional nurse through careful and enthusiastic scholarship. The Christian worldview serves as a framework for the program and the integration of personal faith and learning is encouraged. Students are invited throughout the program to become aware of the paradigms that influence their lives and nursing practice and to make alterations in those paradigms upon careful reflection. The graduate of the program is a generalist, prepared to serve in a variety of settings and to enter graduate level education." The program's Statement of Belief was based on five pillars: the Human Experience, the Discipline of Nursing, Professional Nursing, Health, and Adult Learner.

Further, the RN-to-BSN Korean Nurse Program had a curriculum consisting of four terms and that included classes such as college writing, study of the novel, and short fictions in English, as well as language laboratory, and English classes. Korean wasn't allowed to be spoken in these classes.

Admission into the RN-to-BSN Korean Nurse Program required the following:

- A completed and signed Application for Admission
- A diploma from an accredited Korean nursing school
- An RN licensure based on successful performance on the National Council Licensure Examination (NCLEX)
- Evidence of academic proficiency based on college or postsecondary transcripts and two professional recommendations
- Intermediate-level English skills as determined by an interview at Eastern University or the National Medical Center in Seoul, South Korea

Learning about all these requirements, I was glad to see the Korean nurses needed to have stronger English skills than what I had had when I came to the United States as a nurse. They had to take entire courses in English directly in the classes, even while they were learning English, I assumed that taking courses in English must be difficult for these Korean nurses although they had support from Eastern University. From my experience, learning English was much harder than we had anticipated.

Truly, I hoped these requirements would help Korean nurses with the language barrier or communication since English would be essential for their performance in nursing practice. I was happy that their situation was better than mine and they wouldn't have to go through what I had been through. But I wondered how much it might help them because learning English was not easy, simple, or quick. Particularly when I was stressed, the learning process took much more time.

Since there was a shortage of nurses in the United States, the intensive program, which admitted a new cohort twice a year, helped Korean nurses obtain their degree and secure a job within six months. In each new cohort, the number of students, their ages and gender, and experiences in nursing were different. This was new to me because during my time in nursing school at Ewha Womans College, all my peers were about the same age except for me. Therefore, by the class or year, such as freshman, sophomore, junior, or senior, anyone could figure out the age of the students. But unlike at Ewha, I saw these students were mixed with different looks: some were single and some were with family; some were young and some were old. The only commonality was that they were all nurses; still, they had different levels of experience in nursing in Korea. It reminded me that when I came to America, we were required have a nursing license, be a registered nurse, and have two years of experience in the nursing field, whether we worked in a hospital, a health center, or a school. These requirements are still in place. I hoped these Korean nurses were not the same as I with my English language problems and the need to understand the different culture in America. But I feared that they might have similar problems. With these thoughts in mind, I felt somehow that I had a responsibility to help them. Given my own experiences, I had something to offer. They should not have to go through what I did.

When I began teaching, there were two mixed cohorts of students who struggled with English despite obtaining the NCLEX in English from Korea as part of the program's admission requirements. In addition, they underwent an interview with Eastern University to test their English skills. Cohort 2 had to repeat classes with cohort 3 to overcome the language barrier. This situation clearly indicated that learning English was not easy, just like I had experienced. Their ages ranged from 23 to 58, and there was one male student, which surprised me. Historically, nurses worldwide were typically female, and even in Korea, male nurses would be mocked, but one male nurse was in the class, giving me a clue that the current situation in nursing in Korea had changed since I'd left.

When I learned of this offer to instruct these nurses to obtain their BSN, I thought this must be God's mercy for me because I wanted to be a helper to guide them, asking for what my responsibility and support for them could be. The answers were for sharing and comforting them with all my experiences and struggles that I had faced. I immediately recalled how challenging and demanding the language barrier and cultural differences were for me as I became a nurse in the United States. Then I wondered about these students' experiences navigating the application process in English, what it was like since I left Korea, because I worried that their nursing school's curriculum, where they obtained a diploma nursing degree and spent most of their time in clinical practice, weren't as focused on theory like American nursing school programs. In addition, I was concerned that they were still deeply influenced by Confucianism and thus narrow-minded, focused on the social class differences, which was almost opposite from the American way of thinking. To acclimate to American culture, these nurses would probably struggle like me because the changes or transformation would not happen overnight despite the urgent need. Then my thoughts alerted me that the times have changed, and the living conditions in the same historical background were not the same as when I was in Korea almost 25 years ago. Since I moved away, there had been massive changes to the economy, educational system, and social environment, which could have impacted nursing education. I felt that this would be a good opportunity to observe the differences between them and me as Korean nurses adjusting to life in the United States in comparing my own journey with no support at all. With increased interest, I had more desire to help them from the diploma to obtaining the BSN degree. The result would be win-win for both of us.

Giving thanks to God, I happily accepted this position. There were some losses in practical matters, including a lower salary and a more arduous commute in traffic on the highway from Princeton to Eastern University's main campus in St. Davids, Pennsylvania. But I did not mind at all because I felt that teaching here would be my dream, especially after all my triumphs and my positive experience at Merwick. I had survived three wars—World War II, the Korean War, and the Vietnam War—and had obtained my BSN-RN license from the State Board Examination in Washington, D.C., in 1974, all on my own—without a program like Eastern University's. Most recently, thanks to Merwick, I gained a new appreciation for being a nurse and now had a larger view of nursing as a healer of human life. I was thankful to choose the harder side than the easy side even if it involved heavy challenges. In this direction, I felt that I was moving up to where I wanted to go. That direction was not easy for me, but I made it. If any one of these nurses had a similar background to mine, then I felt this would be perfect for all of us.

But one hesitation was my age. At 66 years old, I was not young anymore. Traditionally, old age made it more difficult to remember things and get around, but my case was different than the traditional way of thinking. Personally, I felt that I was becoming stronger and clearer, and I had more passion for learning than ever before the older I grew. My depth of understanding and my ability to memorize,

VII—Mother, Grandmother, Sister, Counselor, Teacher, Nurse

comprehend, and think and reflect critically on nursing were more enhanced now at 66. With this new dynamic, I was fully confident in myself as a nurse. I wanted to make the Korean nursing students understand my new views, which were fueled by Florence Nightingale and my own experience as a dedicated professional nurse, as opposed to the old concept of nursing. I thought, "It is time to reflect on my transformation in nursing philosophy and my dedication, and I feel an obligation to help these students achieve their goals."

I assessed the causes behind why they became a nurse in Korea and came to the United States, which looked different than mine because of the changed living condition as well as societal aspects. I hoped their reputation was not the same as what I had, the old concept of being a doctor's helper or housemaid. Also, they had already obtained the NCLEX in English in Korea, which was not easy to do, even in the United States as a native English speaker. Passing the NCLEX could be a clear indication of their English proficiency as well as their nursing knowledge. But I discovered that in general, the nurse's salary remained at the same level, and the reputation of a nurse had not changed much over time. Their reasons for becoming a nurse were not much different than mine. I found out that my expectations were not right. Consequently, I figured out that they had to learn more about what nursing was and what nursing was about as a profession.

My teaching subjects were various: holistic nursing, Christian nursing ethics, senior seminar/practicum, and Christian perspective capstone, among others. For the BSN level, these subjects were mandatory, and the students had never studied such topics in Korea in nursing school. When signing up for classes, I found that they had a hard time understanding the course descriptions relating to the objectives, including the requirement of writing a paper at the end of the course. At first, they were unable to read the English textbook because of their problems involving many elements, including a lack of comprehension. Their English was not good enough to read or write at the level where they must be. Although they took all required English courses at Eastern University, still they had many more frustrations and struggles with English problems. I hoped I would be able to help them raise their English-language ability.

I remembered how I had had no help when I was a visiting nurse in Washington, D.C., but how I had eventually been able to overcome my deficiencies. I was not an English teacher obviously, but I was able to explain to them what their problem was because I'd had the same problem. While they needed time to learn it, psychologically I was able to support them and comfort them by sharing my experiences. Otherwise, they would be more nervous and anxious about not being able to comprehend what they were learning. Then I asked them why they wanted to be a BSN in America, and their answers were a little different than mine had been; but many of them had a sense of inferiority for being a nurse, just as I had in Korea. They felt that with a BSN, their reputation could be different, and they wanted to be promoted to higher levels in nursing. Then I asked what was different between their diploma and BSN. They were not sure about what the requirement was, but they knew there must be something different. Whether they knew or not what was important about the BSN, they all wanted to have their BSN badly.

Now I understood well why they wanted to come to the United States like I did; they had almost the same reasons. This led me to think and to study because nursing had not changed in that long period in Korea. That the status of nurses had not changed was quite upsetting. From my observations, I assumed that cultural influence was such an important factor on human service values and social structure of class ranks. This hypothesis further inspired me to teach these nursing students because I wanted them to overcome their own prejudice like I had. Then, with a clearer sense of what was needed, my teaching goals became more ardent.

Naturally, I assessed my roles in these situations, how to assist them through this complicated situation, a task that would be more difficult than I initially expected. My role as a helper for them changed to multiples roles: teacher, counselor, sister, aunt, mother, grandmother, as well as English tutor. It was a huge privilege to be in this position, especially at my old age which was used in a good way. According to Korean culture, elders were supposed to be respected.

Every single individual had very different problems in English and clinical nursing skills, having no real clinical experience like me because they had just practiced in health centers in Korea. Like me, they had more problems writing, reading, and speaking in English, but

VII—Mother, Grandmother, Sister, Counselor, Teacher, Nurse

they had some assistance from the writing center, which was very beneficial for them. Besides, they needed to develop critical thinking skills because they had never been exposed to this way of study. The way they had learned in Korea was to memorize everything. For them, it was not easy to create, criticize, or think independently. Less talking and less questioning was treated as a beauty based on the old culture.

The most common student problems remained English competence and adjusting in different cultural ways. As I mentioned about the requirement of English lessons from Eastern University, they still have major problems comprehending English textbooks. It was new to them to read in English, writing papers, giving case study and current presentations, and fully participating in seminars. When they opened the books, they did not know where to look or what to read because they were not able to comprehend the content. They said that often they became confused and overwhelmed. As a result, they frequently gave up. These descriptions reminded me of exactly the same problems that I used to have when I came to the United States. With that experience, I understood what they were saying, and I was able to share my feelings with them.

They were not able to explain to the American professors what their feelings and problems were because their English ability was not yet good enough. When they attempted to speak with their professors about these matters, the professors were uncertain what they wanted. They tried to understand, but in addition to the language problems, they had not previously taught Korean students and did not understand the cultural differences, just as the Korean students had difficulty comprehending American cultural values. Therefore, the students often became confused and felt overwhelmed by the pressure. Sometimes they lost interest in even trying to read English textbooks. In Korea, they were more used to memorizing what the professors said, and no questions were asked.

To help these students, I reminded them about my past difficulties and how I had endured without the help they were getting from Eastern University. After discussions about this, many of the students felt relieved; they believed now that if I had succeeded in even worse circumstances, they could, too, and that they were fortunate to be at Eastern University which offered assistance to them.

From North Korea to America Through Three Wars

I continued to share my methods for learning English and provided some comfort and confidence to the students. I acted like an English teacher, providing them with emotional support. And many of them began to learn what they needed more quickly, like the differences between English and Korean structure and grammar. They came to understand that they needed to do more than just memorize what their teachers told them. Moreover, gradually they became more aware of the differences between Korean and American culture and were able to adapt in this new society. Many of them told me that my work with them had been really helpful, and I was very pleased about this.

One of the more interesting cultural differences that the students had to learn was eye contact. When to make eye contact and when not to and with whom is an integral part of Korean culture, especially during conversation. Yet in the United States, eye contact is always expected, which is quite the opposite from what I and the nurses had learned growing up. One day, I received a report from the manager where these students had clinical practicum, saying that one Korean nursing student did not pay attention to her during a conversation because she did not maintain eye contact. I explained to this manager about the Korean cultural way of talking. For Koreans, not making eye contact was a form of respect. Now that the manager understood that the student was in fact paying attention and even showing respect, we all laughed and became closer. The communication skills were emphasized based on the American way of showing confidence rather than timidity. Additionally, that they should be ready to ask questions and answer questions naturally was quite new to them. It took time to change because they had to have courage. Keeping multiple roles in general, I emphasized to these students that they were completing the course not just to learn the content but also to help each other, support each other, comfort each other, and be patient, which was quite new to them.

My advice for them was to understand this new way of thinking in the United States. They appreciated me because they were comfortably able to express their mind, feelings, pains, emotions, and family problems between husband and wife. There was more, depending on their individual situation. Through this process, they started to trust me

VII—Mother, Grandmother, Sister, Counselor, Teacher, Nurse

and gained hope from my own experiences. In this situation, thankfully, I reinforced the idea that my age fit well—feeling as a counselor, I said to them, "See what I did. Why can't you do it?" because they knew my situation was worse than theirs. Seeing me now, they were inspired and had more motivation, saying, "Yes, I can do it, too." Also, I encouraged them to help each other, which was somewhat new to them because culturally in Korea, competition tended to limit helping others. One expression of the American way that I liked to share with them was, "Can I help you?" Another one was, "Is there anything that I can do for you?" Whenever I heard expressions like these, I was very impressed. I took them to indicate that cooperation and assistance outweighed competition. They provided a wonderful way to solve problems. In addition, these expressions were used without regard to age, gender, or class. Their use suggested that helping others was part of the larger culture and one that was to be celebrated. Later, they helped each other with a problem. In addition, it was said to everyone regardless of age, gender, and class. I felt that this kind of cultural custom needed everyone in our society helping each other, meaning in a way of humanity.

This instruction significantly applied to one particularly older student among her peers, who felt like a fool in class because she was a slower learner, confused, and often incorrect despite trying her best. She felt that she lost her respect as an elder, which she used to have in Korea. She didn't think she could continue this course because her study demands were becoming heavier every day. I was well suited to show her my whole self and sharing my own situation, from my time at Ewha in Korea up until now in the United States. Gradually, with emotional support and feeling comforted by my own experience, she realized she was in a better position to succeed, and she progressed in her classes. Finally, she completed all the courses. Now she's comfortably practicing as a nurse in America.

Then, one older female student who had been in West Germany for a long time as a nurse, explained the reason why she had enrolled in Eastern University for the BSN program. While in Korea it had been her dream to obtain her BSN in the United States. So, with her strong motivation for obtaining a BSN, she had huge problems with English because she couldn't overcome her traditional way of thinking to critical thinking as well as logical analytical thinking. These concepts were totally new to her. In contrast, there was a young nurse who did not have much nursing experience, so she had less confidence in her studies. At first, she had wanted to be a medical doctor in Korea, but her scores were not strong enough to allow her to enroll in medical school. Then she had the idea that she could be a nurse in a different way by not being in Korea. At that time, coincidently, she heard about Eastern University's RN-to-BSN program. She thought if she became a BSN in the States, she would be a different nurse avoiding giving beside care to patients, which she disliked the most. In Korea, providing such care was looked down on in society. That was why she came to Eastern University, but as she told me, she found out that "a nurse was a nurse no matter where." The American nurse was not much different than the Korean nurse in the patient's room. Regardless of their ages, in general, I found out that there were only a few nurses who wanted to become a nurse to help patients and improve their own knowledge, but still, they were not so satisfied to be a nurse with lower respect from society. More than half were like me, wanting to be a nurse to make a living and still holding a negative view of nursing like I once had. When they were expressing their feelings of inferiority in my office, often they cried and complained about the treatment from the doctors, some of head nurses, and others. They hoped by obtaining their BSN degree that they would escape from these feelings, but they had difficulties following the courses in English and adjusting because of individual different problems. But I urged them to help and support one another. Finally, they were encouraged and understood how helping one another would help them all to obtain the BSN degree.

 Their desire to obtain the BSN was clear and strong, but it took time for them to understand why the BSN was an important goal to reach in becoming a professional nurse. This was not a simple matter because these students were still deeply tied to the old Eastern way of thinking, which adhered less to critical and independent thinking.

 I felt that it was very important to know about what critical thinking is to become a BSN. Critical thinking is a foundational requirement for a BSN; it's the yolk of the egg. But this was new and strange

VII—Mother, Grandmother, Sister, Counselor, Teacher, Nurse

for them like it had been for me. From this point, I had an obligation to teach them how I learned of it and why it was so hard to understand. I had experienced the difficulties with the way of thinking by Confucianism. Again, culturally and traditionally, Koreans were not very accustomed to asking questions; they carried on their work or duties without much thought.

Among the class members, there were age and experience gaps. I had to use my experience to help them understand what critical thinking is regardless of these differences.

The other problem was a problem that I also had because of the culture and social system in Korea for women and for nurses. Traditionally, there were deeply set roots of Confucianism to obey and carry on the order and duty. Therefore, asking a question and to answer one were not easy for them. In the past, women and nurses including me had not used critical thinking which leads to good rationale with clear meaning. The students did not need to have this way of thinking because they were used to obeying orders from doctors and head nurses, no questions asked.

I asked them how they had practiced nursing in the past in Korea. Another question was what were the differences from past and now that they see? What was their nursing history in Korea? What were they learning now? If they found something in a patient, how did they explain that? How did they feel about it? How did this relate to full humanity? Through review of these questions, what meanings did they get?

What I found out was, in general, they were never asked these questions while they were practicing in the past. I was not surprised because I was the same. Then I began to ask them about how and why they make kimchi and rice, which they were eating every day without question. This was a real example. I asked them why they made kimchi, and they had never thought about it. Did they all make kimchi the same way? How did they learn to make it? What's the best way to make kimchi? They all laughed because they all made kimchi, and even rice, in slightly different ways that were learned through family recipes and trial and error. With these examples, they finally grasped the concept of analysis and the importance of questioning. A few students commented that they discovered that they were already thinking critically but not using the same language or definition of critical thinking. They were unaware that they were using critical thinking skills every day—just never in the context of nursing.

I hoped it was a good thing to ask and review how all nurses, East and West, practiced in the past. Should they go back to the past or not? Then, from here they would know where they should go, how they should be as nurses. This whole process of thinking through questions led them to be critical thinkers who could identify, analyze, evaluate, draw, and bring about good results.

Critical thinking would allow them to be creative and independent and develop their own nursing knowledge which was core for the profession. Through this method, they would be able reevaluate their previous notions of nursing to obtain a BSN. This is why critical thinking is so important for professional nursing. When they reached this point, their understanding of nursing would be different than in the past. In turn, they would be enlightened to a new way of nursing that promotes independence and self-confidence and, most important, values human life and seeks to promote the well-being of all individuals in the world.

Nursing is neither new nor old because it has been around since the beginning of human history. There was always a need to provide care. Nursing is a living matter, performed by hands with a deep, caring heart, sometimes through tears when a patient doesn't recover and sometimes through laughter when a patient recovered. But the perception of nursing depended on how people valued nurses throughout history. Nurses weren't always treated highly in the past, regardless of East or West. I did not realize the value and merit of nursing because I never thought critically about nursing. I was prejudiced toward nursing because of my background. But I grew to understand nursing in a way like Florence Nightingale. She just gave nursing care to the people who needed care. Like her, all nurses should be healers of all sorts with caring minds and hearts for the sick, the family and community, and for the whole world.

I was glad that I had an opportunity to demonstrate to these Korean nursing students how my views had changed. With a simplistic view about nursing, I had never asked whether nursing had a history or not, like the Korean students did. I was one of the stereotypes of a

VII—Mother, Grandmother, Sister, Counselor, Teacher, Nurse

Korean nurse obedient to the doctor's order without thought. By doing this, I thought I was a good nurse.

I also explained to them why I went to Villanova University to study gerontological nursing. I told them that it was difficult in the classes and how hard it was for me, just as it was for them, to learn English and read classical and European literature. With these experiences, I had more reasons to understand the Korean students at Eastern University. At that time, I discovered that nursing had a theory like other professions. Nursing theory was difficult for me to understand; even though I loved learning it, the theory took me time to comprehend. My desire to learn nursing theory never stopped despite how hard it was to grasp. This was a transformation, and I developed a new appreciation for being a nurse. The profession of nursing was defined not by being a maid or helper of doctors but based on one's values and desire to help. I had such a negative view of nursing because my interpretation of nursing had been wrong and prejudiced, unlike Florence Nightingale. I told the students that I hoped they all were like me, having the same feelings of appreciation for being a nurse.

At this point, I had a different value and perspective on nursing, which I used to encourage the students to continue their pursuit of the BSN and who would become leaders in the profession. Being a leader, the nursing students would be required to take the courses on nursing ethics, along with the study of holistic nursing, senior seminar, research, leadership and management, and more to help them develop their own theories on nursing. I acknowledged that I had misbehaved for a long time, and because of my limited understanding of the nursing profession, I wasted a lot of time. But over time, I changed, and my hope was that my experience would be helpful to them and they would be glad that they enrolled in this program. By understanding the reasons why they had to take so many courses, they came to understand that they were fortunate to have been able to study these subjects even though they were sometimes difficult courses. A few students told me that they wished they loved to repeat the courses. We all laughed.

Looking back on the experience of the Korean nurses at Eastern University, I was touched by how they studied hard and overcame many obstacles. Sometimes they had to skip their simple supper of ramen soup to prepare for a class presentation. They often were tired and hungry, but they made it. Their verbal skills improved, and they began to use critical thinking and analytical thinking. They now understood and realized the differences between the nursing professions in the United States and Korea. As a result, they came to appreciate their work in the Eastern University RN-BSN program. Now they felt that they were ready to enjoy their new careers and were proud of their BSN degrees and understood why this title was actually useful for a nursing profession. Many of them became nurse practitioners, school nurses, and managers at hospitals, and others continued their education aiming for their doctorate in nursing. They were all impressed by the nursing theories of Florence Nightingale and my own experiences and learned to think more critically.

All they had accomplished exemplified their perseverance. Now they knew more about the Nightingale Pledge than before, and all became aware of her work and why she was so highly recognized by the *New York Times* upon her death in 1910. And they understood why she was so important. They realized why they had to take all subjects that looked new, strange, and difficult and sometimes felt unrelated to nursing.

Finally, they appreciated Eastern University for having this program for Korean nurses. They paid great respect to the institution that provided them with these good opportunities. Many of them hoped to keep this program with its well-deserved high reputation. Unfortunately, this was not possible because the nurse shortage ended by 2015. Korean nurses were unable to work and were encountering visa issues. I felt it was a great honor and immense privilege that I, a Korean nurse who had moved to America, had the opportunity to teach the Korean nursing students. To help them achieve their goals was one of my greatest achievements in my life. My joy fed me full. I deeply thanked God and my brother Sung Kul for being persistent that I become a nurse. Of course, I thanked Eastern University for educating me in the nursing profession and then allowing me to teach courses. It was my tremendous honor and joy to teach Korean nurses at Eastern University.

Remembering the tears of a nursing assistant when I left Merwick, I dried my tears with my bare hands.

VIII

Final Reflections

On June 19, 2015, I gave the presentation, "What Are the Educational Components of Global Nursing?" at the International Council of Nursing (ICN) in Seoul, South Korea. From June 19 to 23, presenters from 130 different countries participated in the conference. I was amazed to see nurses from all over the world dressed in clothing from their respective cultures. All the nurses were energetic and enthusiastic, meandering about, chatting with others, and sharing their excitement about being in South Korea. At 77 years old, I had just finished teaching at Eastern University, and the conference felt like my retirement ceremony. It was my final lecture but also my first ever lecture because I'd never spoken on the international stage. I was nervous and excited when I presented my PowerPoint because it was my first time presenting to such a large crowd; I was used to speaking in small group settings, like my classroom at Eastern University. During my speech, I discussed the need to improve global nursing because the world was shrinking due to improved communication and transportation. I discovered through a follow-up Q&A session that many nurses agreed there was a need for more research on global nursing considering the changing, narrowing world. After the presentation, which went well, I had mixed feelings and was emotional because this opportunity to speak at a conference would be the last in my life. I was also nervous about delivering the same presentation at Ewha Womans University.

The conference center was gigantic. I couldn't tell I was in Seoul; I thought I was still back in the United States. I was so impressed by all the changes in Seoul since I left, which I didn't expect to see: the buildings, designs, all were a scale more reminiscent of American style. Ewha Womans University had changed, too; the campus was well maintained and looked green, with more trees grown than when I was last there. Through these whole scenes, I recalled the Korean strengths and willpower from the old scenes of our difficult past. How hard they must have worked to set up looking like America! I knew how they used to be: not eating enough, resting enough, or sleeping enough. Now it looked like quite a different scene. This made me ask myself, "What did I do in the past? How have I changed?" I was encouraged to do better as a nurse.

Even though I was a native Korean, I felt like a foreigner among the crowd in my homeland. I let my hair go gray instead of dying it black, which was custom in Korea. A Korean resident even approached me in Seoul and asked me if I were American because of my hair. Through the ICN, I had a big, eye-opening opportunity in the nursing world; it was so much bigger than what I'd thought, with countless nurses from many different nations. At the conference, they were positive, energetic, and eager to learn new things. It was very useful to be around all these nurses.

Before returning to the United States, I gave a special lecture to graduate nursing students at Ewha Womans University on the same subject that I presented on at the ICN. At that time, all the students looked like my grandchildren because all their grandmothers were younger than me. They were amazed that I could speak English so well and even that I was still teaching at my age. In Korea, there was the rule in the school system that anyone over the age of 65 years could no longer teach. As I stood on the stage, I remembered my past at Ewha Womans University, when I was the oldest student in the class at that time. Once again, at 77, I was the oldest, but this time I was happy about it. While visiting my alma mater, I learned that even married women could be students at the university, which wasn't allowed during my time there. With changed policy, curriculum, and subjects of nursing, the students' appearances were very different than I expected, with more westernized styles for haircuts, fashion, and shoes. It was very impressive for me while I was reminiscing about my previous life there.

After returning to my home in Princeton, New Jersey, I reviewed all the textbooks that I'd used to teach the Korean nurses at Eastern University, reflecting on my current situation as a professional nursing

VIII—Final Reflections

educator who spoke before a crowd of international nurses. Then I looked back on my life, how it changed completely when I crossed the DMZ in 1948. I lived through three wars (World War II, the Korean War, and the Vietnam War), lost family members, and I never got to be a normal teenager—it was stolen from me. I wished I had never been born. I had to leave my baby girls behind, the hardest thing I've ever done as a mother. I always regretted taking up nursing and blamed myself for being a nurse because of their treatment in society, their reputation of being like a housemaid, according to the Confucian view. Nursing meant working hard without receiving any recognition from society; that was how it was supposed to be. It was so unfair and made me upset. But in my moment of reflection, I discovered how much I finally understood nursing, the power and importance of bedside care. At this time, I felt that I became a new nurse just like the first day, standing in front of a patient in a nurse's uniform, cap, and white shoes. What I disliked about nursing became what I loved. It was sensational to me, realizing my transformation inside of me like when I had discovered at Villanova University that I'd been so ignorant to what nursing was truly about. I was surprised and ashamed of how insensitive and blind I'd been, not seeing the phenomenal benefits of nursing. The more I realized about nursing, the more I desired to provide nursing care. Nursing care is for life and death which is for all human beings.

One of my more senior friends, Young, in Vancouver, Canada, was suffering from multiple, chronic problems and had private care nurses 24/7. I volunteered to move there to provide personal care for her. It was as if I were a novice nurse again. My heart full of empathy, I flew to Vancouver to care for my friend as I should have done sincerely for every patient from the beginning as a nurse. She, a retired statistics professor at the University of British Columbia, and I discussed what nursing was about based on her experiences by me. We talked about what nursing history was in the past: West and East as well as in Korea. She learned the importance of nursing care and the meaning of professional nursing. She was happy to know that nursing was recognized as a profession like statistics. Now it was more highly respected. Also, we admitted that nursing care provided quality of life and dignity to a human being, especially to the elderly. Through our conversations, Young felt very comfortable and peaceful at the end of her life. With this chance to practice again as a nurse, I was reanimated and renewed. When I heard that she had passed away, I was relieved and realized that I'd provided her care until the end. Before she passed, she told her children that she was happy to have a nurse like me at her side. Her children shared this with me.

Always seeking to improve my English, I started to take courses in American literature and American history, and I watched old American movies from the 1950s and 1960s, listened to rock and roll—I didn't even know Elvis Presley's name—and devoured the daily news. While I was listening to rock and roll, I had an experience that I had never had in my life. I was astonished and moved by listening to songs by Elvis Presley, Tina Turner, Harry Belafonte, and others. Their songs were not like an aria by opera singers whom I used to listen to: Maria Callas, Luciano Pavarotti, Plácido Domingo, and so on. They were totally different with their sounds and body movements and songs unlike rock and roll. For classical music, at least, I needed to have some kind of knowledge of the music story and singers to understand and enjoy it. In contrast, for rock and roll I did not need to have any specific knowledge of the songs and singers because I was able to understand the joy, the sorrow, and the hope simply, directly, and quickly while I was listening to them. It was more moving, impressionable, and powerful. It hit me like a home run. I was amazed by the way I felt from them because I had never had a chance to listen to rock and roll in the past. Often, not knowing about rock and roll, I thought this genre was for other people who were very much modernized and westernized. However, music has strong power to move human emotions depending on where, when, and who sang a song that very much related with all humans. With emotional feeling, we laugh and cry, which is essential for our daily living. For me, whenever I hear "Home, Sweet Home" by Sir Henry Rowley Bishop, I think back to Pyeongyang in 1948. I always remember the old memories and cry thinking of that time and circumstance. There was nothing like music for getting back old memories. I even learned about how music has strong relationships with nursing, culture, and literature as well as others. In nursing, music is taking an important place in patient care.

Again, I had a good chance to open my eyes by listening to rock

VIII—Final Reflections

and roll which taught me how much I had been prejudiced in the past. I rejoiced in being awakened and having in some way a new life. With more opened eyes, I was able to pay attention to the singer's body movement, hands, and even fingers, as well as their legs and voice, which is not the traditional way of understanding music. I felt like I was a newborn and seeing a new world in old age. All of this change was a result of continuing to learn English and continuing to learn about nursing and myself.

In addition, I found out through watching the daily news that there was another discovery that I had not yet realized. All the connections with news, music, and literature in the world showed me that life has always been connected from one to another. Until I realized this perspective, I was thinking about each subject independently. It took a long time for me to sense and understand the multiple connections. I felt that my life was becoming rich inside of me and full of energy to be positive despite the problems of aging at the same time. The values of human history, literature, religion, science, politics, and more appealed to my new values and perception. I felt clearly about these new values and perspectives, which made my attitude change toward creativity and a deeper understanding of how much they all were important in our human existence. In fact, it has always been that way, but I just learned it with a new heart. Consequently, I felt my own life was also connected to this meaning of life. My life story could have a meaning in this complicated and complex real world.

For a long time, I wanted to write a memoir, but I didn't feel ready yet. Also, I didn't feel courageous or wise enough to tell my story. But around two years ago, when I was living in Palm Springs, California, I met Lynn Hamilton, a retired U.S. Army nurse, at my Presbyterian church, and she encouraged me to write a few paragraphs about my experience in Vietnam. Lynn had served in Japan and wanted to know about my time in Vietnam; she was surprised I'd worked there as a Korean civilian nurse. She shared this fact about me with her relative, Kenton Clymer, PhD, a retired professor of history at Northern Illinois University, which piqued his interest. He'd studied American relations with Southeast Asia but was unfamiliar with Korean civilians ever going to Vietnam as nurses. Understandably, he had questions for me since this was my experience. He then put me in touch with a Korean scholar at his university, a former student of his, who contacted me to learn about my story as well. I visited my brother Sung Kul in Chicago last year for his 90th birthday and met Kenton's former student, and we became friends. She urged me to write my story, too, but I was still hesitant. I moved from Palm Springs to Pittsburgh, Pennsylvania, where I currently reside, and read Florence Nightingale's biography once again, which had initially inspired me to embrace nursing, but this time, it also encouraged me to write about my own story.

Now, in today's complicated world with Covid-19, war, and terror that is rapidly changing with new technology, I write this book for future nurses who will be in a more difficult situation than I was because the demands and needs for nurses are increasing along with huge social problems and newly discovered diseases. Being a nurse is not easy. It's hard physically, mentally, and emotionally, with different shifts, day and night, and not having regular holidays off. All of these issues are our challenge in nursing. But if you consider my own experiences, there are plenty of possibilities to be successful as a nurse. My advice is that each individual nurse stands on self-reliance, self-determination, and integrity and remains energetic, innovative, proactive, and hardworking. But most important, nurses need to know what nursing is about: providing nursing care from birth to death. The heart of nursing is the same, whether in war or peace. Nurses need to know what living is and what dying is. Nursing is attached to life

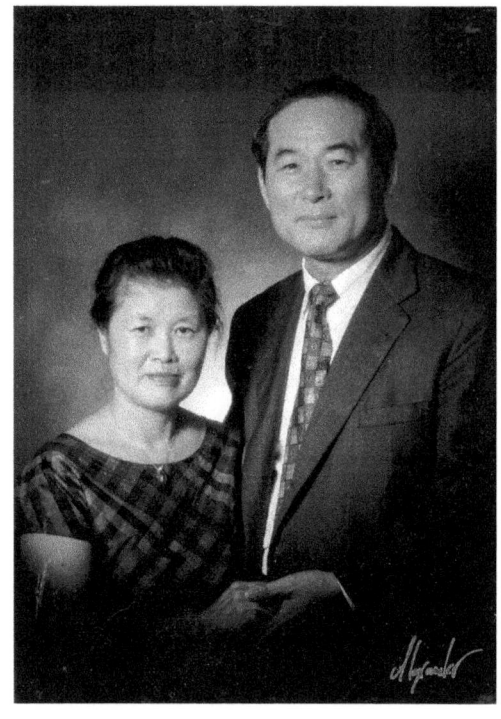

Sung Yoo and Insok Yoo, 1994.

VIII—Final Reflections

from the beginning to the end, regardless of skin color, race, gender, nationality, political belief, age, and place of birth. Nurses are pioneers of human life. We are all nurses in one body, we all live together but in different places like human organs in one body. As a result, we are here for the well-being of all human beings. Remember, nursing makes a new life. To know this value, I spent my whole life, but for future nurses, I hope my experience will provide a useful resource. If I still didn't know the heart of nursing, then I would not be able to share this advice happily. I thank God that He helped me to be transformed so that I could write this memoir. I am happy to be a nurse—this is really an unbelievable and unexpected moment—and I wish all future nurses the same happiness with my deepest sincerity. Remember, you are pioneers of the health of all human beings, and you can build a healthier world. "Keep going forward."

Afterword

Navigating the Historical and Sociopolitical Intersection of Nurse Migration

by HEEYOUNG CHOI

Workforce migration of trained nurses has been a long-standing phenomenon in the health professions.[1] With globalization, the demand for nurses in developed countries has increased steadily, leading to rapid growth in the migration of nurses. Today, there are only a few countries unaffected by nurse migration, and the global phenomenon of nurse migration is becoming a familiar aspect of daily life for millions of patients and caregivers worldwide. A significant number of nurses migrate in search of better salaries, work conditions, opportunities for professional development, improved quality of life, personal safety, or simply new opportunities.[2] The patterns and characteristics of international migration between countries have varied and changed over time. Overall, nurse migration is influenced by a combination of pull-and-push factors, both abroad and domestically, resulting from individual choices. From the perspective of patients and stakeholders involved, nurse migration entails both benefits and challenges—and due to the complex nature of the healthcare landscape, there is no single theoretical framework that can fully explain the comprehensive spectrum of factors influencing nurses' migration decisions.[3]

Traditionally, the pattern of nurse migration involved moving from developing to developed nations. For instance, individuals from

Afterword

the Philippines, India, China, the Caribbeans, and sub-Saharan Africa immigrated to Western countries such as the United Kingdom, United States, Canada, and Australia.[4] South Korea is among the countries that produce and export a significant number of nurses.

The United States is unquestionably the most preferred destination for Korean nurses. As of 2022, approximately 24 million residents of the United States are of Asian descent, with 1.9 million identifying as Korean.[5] Korean Americans constitute the tenth largest immigrant population within the United States and are the fifth largest group among Asian immigrants; they represent one of the fastest growing immigrant communities.[6] Nurses rank among the predominant occupational groups among Korean immigrants, particularly among female immigrants. According to the South Korean Ministry of Health and Welfare, the number of Korean nurses preparing to immigrate to the United States reached 8,350 in 2022 and 2023 combined.[7]

This situation is quite different from the 1960s, when the Korean government and local authorities promoted overseas migration. Nevertheless, the number of Korean nurses taking the U.S. National Council Licensure Examination for Registered Nurses (NCLEX-RN) has continued to increase. According to recent studies[8] on the intent of Korean nursing students to migrate abroad, economic reasons remain a major factor for the migration of Korean nurses and nursing students. Additionally, professional development and career opportunities are another reason why nursing students are interested in migration. Korean nurses often express dissatisfaction with how the nursing profession is treated in Korean society. In particular, the unequal relationship between doctors and nurses as well as the attitudes of patients stemming from patriarchal traditions have shown to contribute toward low self-esteem among Korean nurses. Korean nurses decide to migrate for professional development not offered in Korea, anticipating better compensation and a professional career. Personal educational advancement is also a reason for migration. Nurses who plan to return to their home country in the future often seek advanced degrees, including a PhD, as a valuable asset after migrating. In a few cases, some nursing students wish to migrate due to political and social instability in Korea. For example, concerns about political instability, such as the possibility of war between

North and South Korea, have led them to decide on migration as a contingency plan.

Among noneconomic reasons, the status of women or family values are also cited. Although Korean culture is undergoing significant changes, conservative Confucian ideals are still deeply rooted in Korean society, imposing heavy burdens of professional and domestic responsibilities on women. From this perspective, Korean nurses, who are predominantly female, choose to migrate in hopes of finding a less restricted life as women and greater personal freedom in Western countries. Some choose to migrate to raise and educate their children in a different educational environment. They use their nursing qualifications to cover the costs of their children's education in foreign countries which provide a less competitive educational environment compared with Korea. English-speaking countries are the most preferred destinations for migration, with the United States remaining the unequivocal favorite for nursing students or nurses.

Within these contexts, the story of Sung C. Yoo exemplifies the immigration of Korean nurses to the United States. It is also important to note, however, that she is not merely an example of a nurse migrating from Korea to the United States. Yoo's life journey involved incessantly crossing territorial boundaries, whether by choice or by necessity, amid the backdrop of World War II, the Korean War, and the Vietnam War. The most notable aspect is that Yoo was born in present-day North Korea and lived a comfortable life there until fleeing with her mother to the southern part of the Korean peninsula at a young age, escaping persecution by the communist regime following the end of World War II and Korea's liberation. In other words, she was a *wŏllammin*, those who migrated from today's North Korea to South Korea and eventually acquired citizenship from the Republic of Korea (ROK).[9] The term *wŏllammin* used here specifically refers to those who crossed from North to South Korea from the time immediately following liberation from Japan through the Korean War period (1945–1953). Yoo was also among the graduates of early nursing bachelor's programs in Korea. She had firsthand experience in nursing education and health profession programs established under ROK's nation-building projects after its liberation from Japan. Furthermore, she notably migrated to Vietnam to undertake nursing duties as part

Afterword

of a South Korean civilian medical team whose pay and benefits were directly provided by the U.S. government during the Vietnam War. And shortly after returning to Korea, she emigrated to the United States.

Migration is fundamentally understood as a multifaceted process of individuals crossing boundaries. This process includes the flow of people, goods, services, images, and ideas across boundaries. The tumultuous life of Yoo, as depicted in *From North Korea to America Through Three Wars*, illustrates the shifting and evolving boundaries of nation, ethnicity, class, and gender perceptions as individuals traverse territorial and national boundaries. Yoo experienced a constant transformation of her perceived identity boundaries, being the daughter of a socially and economically privileged family from North Korea; a *wŏllammin* who faced persecution and discrimination while living in the south; a nurse, one of the professions not respected in Korea; a medical professional who could gain economic benefits from participating in the Vietnam War; a Korean woman who experienced Western education and culture earlier than other Koreans; and an immigrant who struggled with language barriers despite finding satisfaction through the "democratic" experiences in the United States. Yoo's memoir candidly describes these processes in a quite detailed manner, allowing readers to immerse themselves in the vivid experiences of a woman from North Korea.

From North Korea to America Through Three Wars encompasses a diverse range of themes including healthcare, war, immigration, and women's experiences. It chronicles Yoo's life journey starting from her childhood in North Korea, her migration to the southern part of the Korean peninsula after liberation, seeking refuge in the southern regions during the Korean War, working as a nurse in Vietnam, and finally emigrating and settling in the United States. Particularly noteworthy is the inclusion of stories that have not been properly discussed in the discourse of modern Korean history, making Yoo's memoir valuable for future research and educational texts.

More specifically, the memoir portrays aspects such as the lives of *wŏllammin* who settled in Seoul before and after the Korean War, the public perception of nursing education and nursing duties in Korea during the 1950s and 1960s, the experiences of female nurses within

South Korean civilian medical teams participating in the Vietnam War, and the nature of nursing work, professional beliefs, and identity changes within the United States. Thus, it provides various perspectives and insights for conducting research examining the impact of nation-building projects carried out under the slogan of liberation from Japanese colonial rule in Korea and their influence on individuals. In summary, Yoo's memoir serves as a rich source material for scholarly discourse on *wŏllammin*, Korean medical history, and nurse immigration, offering diverse viewpoints and implications for examining the projects undertaken under the nation-building slogan in postliberation Korea and their impact on individuals.

The major events in Yoo's life journey described in *From North Korea to America Through Three Wars* are closely connected to research in modern Korean history. Regarding the *wŏllammin* before the outbreak of the Korean War, Korean historians such as Kang Jung-Koo and Kim Kwi-ok have discussed their origins, the intentions behind their migration, and the challenges they faced in settling down shortly after liberation.[10] According to this research, the scale of *wŏllammin* migrating southward due to land reforms and religious repression in North Korea since the mid–1946 had already surpassed 400,000 by the end of the same year, with the majority fleeing for political and ideological reasons. Especially after the decision of the Moscow Conference in December 1945, there was a significant influx of *wŏllammin*, particularly Christians and right-wing nationalists, and the housing issues deteriorated in Seoul. The life of Yoo's family serves as a historical record, illustrating how North Koreans, predominantly right-wing Christians from Pyongan Province and holding landlord power, adapted to life in Seoul after fleeing. This topic had previously been explored to only a limited extent through demographic studies. Yoo's description of her migration and refugee experience as a girl under ten years old in *From North Korea to America Through Three Wars* provides a deep understanding of how the influx of *wŏllammin* affected the Seoul community, how their settlement unfolded within the local context of Seoul, and sheds light on another journey of hardship triggered by the outbreak of the Korean War.

For a comprehensive understanding of the establishment of the 20th-century nursing education system in Korea and the participation

Afterword

of Korean female medical professionals in the Vietnam War, the book *Reconstructing Bodies: Biomedicine, Health, and Nation-Building in South Korea Since 1945* by John DiMoia serves as a valuable resource for delving into the topics that comprise more than half of *From North Korea to America Through Three Wars*, providing insights into the historical context and developments within the Korean healthcare system.[11] *Reconstructing Bodies* explores key themes related to the gradual transition from German and Japanese medical knowledge to American and international medical models, as well as various forms of private organization intervention and adaptation, and the adoption of a government-led health management model within the anti-communist regime in postliberation Korea. Organized along historical lines, six case studies in medical and health-related topics are presented to elucidate different themes. DiMoia emphasizes that South Korea's series of choices from 1945 to the present regarding biomedical practices were deeply imbued with ideological dimensions similar to those in North Korea. He further argues that although each choice proved successful in its own right, South Korea's decision to embrace biomedical culture was, in reality, the result of a deeply ambivalent and unstable process characterized by profound ambivalence.[12] DiMoia's research into the establishment of the healthcare education and public health system in Korea under the guise of anti-communist nation-building, as well as the reality of medical projects executed under the influence of the United States, provides background information for Yoo's journey of obtaining nursing qualifications and becoming an experienced nurse through the process of immigration.

To understand Yoo's experience of working in Vietnam for one year as a nurse belonging to a civilian medical team, it is necessary to pay attention to recent studies on the participation of South Korean military nurses in the Vietnam War. First, in the 2005 paper, Ji Yeon-ok categorized the experiences of six former South Korean military nurse officers who participated in the Vietnam War.[13] According to this study, the military nurse officers were deployed overseas with determination to enhance national prestige and a deep love for their country. They encountered various situations they had not experienced before and gained new experiences. Moreover, they completed their missions with strong mental resilience, endured everything, and felt a camaraderie akin to brotherhood, especially toward their male counterparts in the South Korean military. They took pride in fulfilling their duty as part of history. In 2016 and 2019, Han Jeong-jin's papers conducted a more in-depth analysis of the content revealed by Ji Yeon-ok's interviews. Han interviewed 14 female military nurse officers who participated in the Vietnam War from 1964 to 1973 and analyzed an analysis of artworks related to the war.[14] The study particularly argued new facts, such as the ability of female nurse officers, who were a minority serving as noncombatants in predominantly male combat zones, to empathize with the war wounds experienced by local women and to realize the constraints faced by female nurse officers. At times, they even protested against irrational discrimination. The nurse officers highlighted in these studies were affiliated with the South Korean military, which differs in background and status from Yoo's experience as a civilian medical worker. However, as Korean women undertaking nursing duties during wartime, their experiences are considered important research subjects for analyzing Yoo's experiences through a gender lens.

Indeed, research on the emigration of Asian professionals to the United States and other Western countries can be valuable for understanding the immigration background of Korean nurses like Yoo.[15] Existing studies on Asian American immigrants have emphasized the shortage of nursing personnel in the United States since World War II, attributing to the Immigration and Nationality Act of 1965, which allocated visas to needed skilled workers. Some studies have explained the phenomenon of immigration in professional fields, including nursing, using the economic logic of "brain drain."[16] According to the "brain drain" theory, the failure of Asian countries to provide professional and economic opportunities commensurate with their skills and training has prompted many Asian professionals to migrate to the United States in pursuit of economic opportunities.

The history of Filipino nurses emigrating to the United States has been actively explored, given that Filipino nurses outnumber other Asian groups.[17] Among these, Catherine Ceniza Choy's *Empire of Care: Nursing and Migration in Filipino American History*[18] challenged existing research that grouped Filipino nurse immigrants

Afterword

with other Asian nations or other professional migrants from the Philippines. More specifically, Choy aimed to understand and evaluate immigrants as multifaceted historical subjects, challenging the prevailing notion that the migration of modern Filipino nurses was merely a pursuit of economic gain. Instead, Choy's analysis, which focuses on the notable history and culture between the Philippines and the United States, enables a deeper understanding of the motivations for Filipino nurses' migration and how perceptions of America in 20th-century Asia influenced their decisions. She points out that it is not simply economic benefits but also a complex set of factors supporting migration to the United States, such as the U.S. government, immigrant recruitment agencies, professional nursing organizations in the Philippines, and networks of Filipino nurse migrants. The cultural aspects of Filipino nursing education and migration emphasized in *Empire of Care* provide valuable information for comparative analysis with other ethnic or racial groups of nurses when examining various cultural experiences mentioned in Yoo's memoir.

Yoo, who has lived in the United States since 1971, generally felt satisfied with her life despite facing language barriers. This was especially true in her nursing profession—this leads to the question of whether other groups of Korean immigrants might have experienced similar sentiments. Two specific groups provide analogous examples: first, Korean nurse immigrants who primarily settled in Germany before moving to the United States; second, Korean immigrants who were predominantly engaged in small businesses in the United States during the same period. For more information on the former group, Yong-Suk Jung's "Beyond the Bifurcated Myth" is recommended, and for the latter, *On My Own: Korean Businesses and Race Relations in America* by In-Jin Yoon provides in-depth insights.[19]

According to Jung's research, nurses or nurse aides who emigrated to Germany during the same period had generally unsatisfactory experiences as immigrants, leading to a lack of overall satisfaction.[20] As evidenced by a document found in the archive of the German Hospital Federation (Deutsche Krankenhausgesellschaft), some Korean nurses expressed dissatisfaction with their working environment, living conditions, and contract terms in Germany. Some Korean nurse immigrants were unsuccessful in finding satisfaction in their jobs and complained about unfavorable working conditions, leading to early termination of their contracts. Many of them were assigned to psychiatric hospitals, rural hospitals, and nursing homes requiring intense physical labor, places where many were reluctant to work. Consequently, they frequently sought to avoid these assignments by continuously relocating to different places. Overall, their lives were marked by instability, particularly because any failure to obtain consent from their employers was considered a breach of contract, resulting in immediate termination of their work and residency permits.[21]

As Yoon argued in *On My Own*, Korean immigrants in the 1970s, predominantly small business owners, did not find satisfaction upon emigrating to the United States. Many of them came from educated middle-class backgrounds and had previously held clerical positions in Korea. Some wealthy Korean entrepreneurs or high-ranking government officials and professionals were able to emigrate to the United States on tourist visas. They brought substantial funds from Korea to invest in new businesses in the United States, aiming to obtain permanent residency status under U.S. immigration laws. Their pursuit of small businesses was not necessarily driven by a passion for entrepreneurship.[22] Facing challenges in language communication and unfamiliarity with American culture, they struggled to secure jobs that aligned with their education and career backgrounds in Korea. Consequently, they were compelled to accept their circumstances and settle for reality. Furthermore, the businesses they chose required immense physical, mental, and social costs and sacrifices. Many Korean immigrant small business owners suffered from chronic illnesses and mental disorders across all ages due to long working hours and tremendous stress. Every year, a considerable number of Korean immigrant small business owners were injured or lost their lives at the hands of robbers.[23]

Yoo's memoir does not detail the discriminatory treatment or dissatisfaction that other Korean immigrants have experienced. While acknowledging the significant challenges of overcoming language barriers and passing the American nursing licensure exam, Yoo predominantly reflects a positive outlook. She appreciates the various job opportunities available in the United States, the support she received in the hospital setting, and her experiences of

Afterword

"democracy" in America. In this sense, Yoo's experience cannot be generalized or applied universally to all Korean nurse immigrants or immigrants in general. Research conducted by Jung and Yoon could provide valuable insights into understanding the reasons behind Yoo's relatively high satisfaction compared to others in her immigration experience.

In both Korea and in the United States, there remains a lack of public awareness and personal reflection regarding the contributions of Korean nurse immigrants in America and other countries. While Korean scholars have been conducting research on Korean nurse immigrants within the context of the growing interest in immigration of educated individuals and professionals to the United States, much of this research has focused on specific time periods, regions, or current situations.[24] Although there exist monographs on the history of nursing in Korea, there has been modest attempt to explain the phenomenon of nurse migration from historical and cultural perspectives within the context of Korean nursing education.[25] In the U.S. academic community, there has not been sufficient discussion on the immigration experiences of Korean nurses, making it difficult to understand their relationships with colleagues of different ethnic backgrounds, local residents in the immigration countries, and experiences with healthcare or government administrators. Moreover, there is a lack of research connecting the sociopolitical context, including the impact of wars such as World War II, the Korean War, and the Vietnam War, to the history of Korean nursing migration and immigration. In particular, the participation of Korean women in the Vietnam War has been inadequately addressed.[26] These are why I place high value on *From North Korea to America Through Three Wars*.

I see *From North Korea to America Through Three Wars* as a valuable resource for deepening the existing narratives and conceptions surrounding *wŏllammin*, Korean medical education, participation in the Vietnam War, and immigration to the United States. This is especially pertinent within the historical context of national reconstruction efforts after liberation and the Korean War, spearheaded by the South Korean government. Utilizing *From North Korea to America Through Three Wars* and the aforementioned secondary resources, scholars could develop research projects that expand on the mid- to late 20th-century's medical, war, and cultural history in several impactful ways. Here are a few research ideas.

Uncovering the Historical Context of Korean Nurse Immigration: Scholars could conduct extensive research to understand the historical background of Korean nurses emigrating to Vietnam and the United States, focusing on the context of military rule and national reconstruction in South Korea. This study would involve interviewing individuals who experienced these migrations, providing insight into the formation of the international Korean labor force through the lenses of race, gender, and class. For researchers who particularly would be interested in the story of the medical team deployed to Vietnam, I find that the National Archives of Korea documents titled "P'awŏl ŭiryodan ch'ŏl" (The collection of the medical team deployed to Vietnam) would be helpful.[27] The collection includes résumés, activity records, insurance certificates, and more of the civilian medical team, most of which are accessible to the public upon request on-site. Therefore, researchers would benefit greatly from the archive.

Examining Yoo's Journey as a *Wŏllammin*: I anticipate the emergence of studies that delve into Yoo's personal journey as a *wŏllammin*, who became a graduate of South Korea's nursing bachelor's program, a Korean nurse deployed to the Vietnam War, and a U.S. immigrant, within the broader framework of Korean nursing education and migration during the 1950s–70s. Such analyses would necessitate an examination of whether Yoo and individuals similar to her truly encountered the promised opportunities, equality, and citizenship within South Korea's medical education system and immigration policies of that era, or if they encountered unanticipated obstacles attributable to their unique circumstances. It is noteworthy that *Wŏllammin kusul saengaesa chosa yŏn'gu* (Survey of oral life history of *wŏllammin*) has recently been made available to the public.[28] This is the result of a three-year study supported by the Korea Research Promotion Project, conducted by Professor Kim Seongbo and his research team from the Department of History at Yonsei University. The team engaged with 149 *wŏllammin* over about 150 meetings, recording 100 hours of oral histories. This material, accessible through an online website will be a significant resource for conducting various research

Afterword

topics related to *wŏllammin*, building on the experiences described in Yoo's memoir.

Shifting Perceptions: Yoo's memoir serves as a meaningful catalyst in redirecting attention away from perceiving nurses solely as labor commodities within a single organization, and instead encourages the recognition of nurses as historical actors with distinctive perspectives and life experiences. Consequently, it would be invaluable to explore Korean perceptions of *wŏllammin* and nurses overall, the attitudes of Korean governmental and health authorities, the viewpoints of Korean women who served in the Vietnam War regarding Vietnam and its people, and the perspectives of U.S. government officials and hospital employers towards Korean nurse immigrants. Such an investigation would provide deeper insights into the multifaceted dynamics influencing the migration journeys of Korean nurses and shed light on the broader socio-political contexts within which their experiences unfolded.

Exploring the Legacy of U.S. Imperialism: Yoo's memoir would serve as a valuable tool for critically analyzing the enduring legacies of U.S. imperialism and understanding their impact on individuals, including Koreans and Korean Americans. By engaging with Yoo's narrative, scholars can conduct studies to investigate how these legacies may have influenced the experiences of Korean nurses and Korean immigrants in the United States, particularly regarding issues of identity, citizenship, and belonging. For example, Sung's experience of American people and culture in Vietnam and later in America would show an aspect of South Korea's understated issues reflecting a negative, dark history involving U.S. imperialism.

Prospective research projects incorporating above-mentioned elements could provide a comprehensive and insightful analysis of the migration experiences of Korean nurses, shedding light on their individual stories within the broader historical and sociopolitical contexts of the time. Individual narratives of migration experiences provide valuable insights into the complexity and diversity of migration phenomena. Factors such as economic, social, and political influences, as well as the roles of local authorities and immigration stakeholders and the adaptation of immigrants to society and their interactions with the local community are key topics in migration studies. Yoo's story illustrates various aspects of nurse migration phenomena, shedding light on ongoing regional, economic, and policy-related issues. For these reasons, I expect that scholars in fields such as medicine, war, women's studies, and cultural history, as well as individuals interested in modern history, particularly those working in healthcare, would find Yoo's memoir interesting enough to spark new research and discussions.

The significance of *From North Korea to America Through Three Wars* is further underscored by the ongoing journey of Yoo, who transcends boundaries. As a woman who experienced war, she has now come to proudly share her past with people who differ from her in skin color and background. She has walked a unique path in life, always clinging to her faith in herself and making the most of her decisions, no matter how daunting they were at the time. She has grown to love her life as a woman who endured to the end. Reflecting on her past, she confesses that wherever she went, she felt the guiding hand of the Lord. Her fondness for sharing her favorite Bible verses highlights her desire to emphasize her identity as a Christian beyond being a refugee, a nurse, and an immigrant. She often cites 1 Corinthians 13:7, "There is nothing love cannot face; there is no limit to its faith, its hope, its endurance," confessing that her life has been a testament to a love transcending boundaries. The book concludes with anticipation for her future endeavors that *cross further boundaries* and the potential sequel to *From North Korea to America Through Three Wars*.

Heeyoung Choi *is a visiting scholar in the Department of History at Northern Illinois University and is also an adjunct faculty member at Korea National University of Arts. She completed her training in Korean music theory and history at Seoul National University and the Academy of Korean Studies. Her research interests include diasporic music, traditional Korean music, women's studies, and Asian American cultural studies.*

Chapter Notes

Foreword

1. American Association of Colleges of Nursing, *The Essentials: Core Competencies for Professional Nursing Education* (Washington, D.C.: American Association of Colleges of Nursing, 2021), 49.
2. American Nursing Association, *ANA Nursing: Scope and Standards of Nursing Practice*, 4th ed. (Silver Spring, MD: American Nurses Association, 2021), 2.
3. Jean C. Whelan, "American Nursing: An Introduction to the Past," in "Nursing, History, and Health Care," online in *PennNursing, University of Pennsylvania*, 2011. https://www.nursing.upenn.edu/nhhc/.
4. American Association of Colleges of Nursing, *The Essentials*, 2.
5. Whelan, "American Nursing."
6. Joan E. Lynaugh, "Education," in "Nursing, History, and Health Care," online in *PennNursing, University of Pennsylvania*, 2011. https://www.nursing.upenn.edu/nhhc/education/.
7. Louise C. Selanders, cited in "History Lesson: Nursing Education Has Evolved Over the Decades," *Nurse.com Blog*, November 5, 2012. www.nurse.com/blog/history-lesson-nursing-education-has-evolved-over-the-decades/.
8. Whelan, "American Nursing."
9. News Release, Institute of Medicine, "Linda Aiken, Whose Research Revealed the Importance of Nursing in Patient Outcomes, Receives Institute of Medicine's 2014 Lienhard Award," *Institute of Medicine, National Academies, Washington, D.C.*, October 20, 2014. https://www.nationalacademies.org/news/2014/10/linda-aiken-whose-research-revealed-the-importance-of-nursing-in-patient-outcomes-receives-institute-of-medicines-2014-lienhard-award.
10. Whelan, "American Nursing."
11. Bureau of Labor Statistics, 2023, in Rebecca Munday, "Male Nurse Statistics: A Look at the Numbers," *NurseJournal* (updated March 28, 2024). https://nursejournal.org/articles/male-nurse-statistics/.
12. Whelan, "American Nursing."
13. History.com, "Florence Nightingale's Impact on Nursing," *History.com*, November 9, 2008 (updated April 24, 2023). https://www.history.com/topics/womens-history/florence-nightingale-1#florence-nightingale-s-impact-on-nursing.
14. Whelan, "American Nursing."
15. Patricia D'Antonio, "To Degree or Not to Degree," in "Nursing, History, and Health Care," online in *PennNursing, University of Pennsylvania*, 2011. https://www.nursing.upenn.edu/nhhc/.
16. Linda Laskowski-Jones, "Raising the Bar on Respect for Nursing as a Career," *Nursing2024*, 49 (October 2019): 6. https://journals.lww.com/nursing/Fulltext/2019/10000/Raising_the_bar_on_respect_for_nursing_as_a_career.1.spx.
17. Lynaugh, "Education."
18. Korean International Cooperation Agency, "History of Korea's Overseas Employment and Migration,"

Notes—Introduction

https://artsandculture.google.com/story/vwVRJ0los_GuKA.

19. Pyong Gap Min, in Soojin Chung, "History of Korean Nursing Immigration to American, from 1903 to Present," *Korean Diaspora Project, Boston University School of Theology*. https://sites.bu.edu/koreandiaspora/issues/history-of-korean-immigration-to-america-from-1903-to-present/.

20. Stacey Newton, Jennifer Pillay, and Gina Higginbottom, "The Migration and Transitioning Experiences of Internationally Educated Nurses: A Global Perspective," *Journal of Nursing Management* 20 (2012): 534.

21. Myungsun Yi and Mary Ann Jezewski, "Korean Nurses Adjustment to Hospitals in the United States," *Journal of Advanced Nursing* 32 (2000): 721. [Abstract]

22. Geraldine Bednash in "History Lesson: Nursing Education Has Evolved over the Decades," *Nurse.com Blog*, November 5, 2012. www.nurse.com/blog/history-lesson-nursing-education-has-evolved-over-the-decades/.

23. "ANA Code of Ethics with Interpretive Statements," in American Nurses Association, *Nursing: Scope and Standards of Practice*, 15.

24. American Association of Colleges of Nursing, *The Essentials*, 3.

25. *Ibid.*, 4.

Introduction

1. "DPRK-Russia Treaty on Comprehensive Strategic Partnership," *KCNA Watch*. https://kcnawatch.org/newstream/1718870859-459880358/dprk-russia-treaty-on-comprehensive-strategic-partnership/.

2. Kim Il-sung, "On Progressive Democracy: A Lecture Given to the Students of the Pyongyang Worker-Peasant Political School," October 3, 1945, in *Works*, vol. 1 (Pyongyang: Foreign Language Publishing House, 1980), 254, 267.

3. "The Enemy Within: Shadow of Japanese Past Hangs Over S. Korea," *France24*, July 3, 1919. https://.france24.com/en/20190307-enemy-within-shadow-japanese-past-hangs-over-korea; Choe Sang-Hun, "Colonial-Era Dispute Agitates South Koreans," *New York Times*, April 4, 2010. https://www.nytimes.com/2010/04/05/world/asia/05poet.html. A Truth and Reconciliation Commission was also appointed in December 2005 to investigate not only Japanese collaborators but also people responsible for human rights abuses, massacres, and violent suppression of dissents under the authoritarian regimes of Syngman Rhee, Park Chung-hee, and Chun Doo-hwan.

4. "South Korea Releases Japanese Colonial Collaborator List," *History News Network*, August 29, 2005. https://www.historynewsnetwork.org/article/south-korea-releases-japanese-colonial-collaborato.

5. Sheila Miyoshi Jager, "Korean Collaborators: South Korea's Truth Committees and the Forging of a New Pan-Korean Nationalism," *Asia-Pacific Journal/Japan Focus* 3 (2005). https://apjjf.org/Sheila-Miyoshi-Jager/2170/article.

6. Recommended books about the domestic and international dimensions of the Korean War include Bruce Cumings, *The Origins of the Korean War*, vol. 1, *Liberation and the Emergence of Separate Regimes, 1945–1947* (Princeton: Princeton University Press, 1981), and vol. 2, *The Roaring of the Cataract, 1947–1950* (Princeton: Princeton University Press, 1992); William Stueck, *The Korean War: An International History* (Princeton: Princeton University Press, 1997); William Stueck, ed., *The Korean War in World History* (Lexington: University Press of Kentucky, 2004); William Stueck, *Rethinking the Korean War: A New Diplomatic and Strategic History* (Princeton: Princeton University Press, 2013); Sergei Goncharov, John Lewis, and Xue Litai, *Uncertain Partners: Stalin, Mao, and the Korean War* (Stanford: Stanford University Press, 1993); and Shen Zhihua, *Mao, Stalin and the Korean War: Trilateral Communist Relations in the 1950s*, trans. Neil Silver (London: Routledge, 2012).

Notes—Introduction

7. See Peter Duus, *The Abacus and the Sword: The Japanese Penetration of Korea, 1895–1910* (Berkeley: University of California Press, 1998).

8. See, for instance, Totsuka Etsuro, "Japan's Colonization of Korea in Light of International Law," *Asia-Pacific Journal/Japan Focus* 9 (2011). https://apjjf.org/2011/9/9/totsuka-etsuro/3493/article.

9. On the transformation of Korean society under colonial rule, see Gi-Wook Shin and Michael Robinson, *Colonial Modernity in Korea* (Cambridge, MA: Harvard East Asia Center, 1999); Chan Seung Park, "Japanese Rule and Colonial Dual Society in Korea," *Korea Journal* 50 (2010): 69–98; Hong Yung Lee, Yong-Chool Ha, and Clark W. Sorensen, eds., *Colonial Rule and Social Change in Korea, 1910–1945* (Seattle: University of Washington Press, 2013); and E. Taylor Atkins, "Colonial Modernity," in *Routledge Handbook of Modern Korean History*, ed. Michael Seth (London: Routledge, 2016), 124–140.

10. See Michael A. Schneider, "The Limits of Cultural Rule: Internationalism and Identity in Japanese Responses to Korean Rice," in Shin and Robinson, *Colonial Modernity*, 97–127; Paul S. Nam, "The Immiseration of the Korean Farmer during the Japanese Colonial Period," *Journal of Agrarian Change* 18 (2018): 281–298.

11. Joseph Seeley and Aaron Skabelund, "Tigers—Real and Imagined—in Korea's Physical and Cultural Landscape," *Environmental History* 20 (2015): 475–503.

12. Michael Robinson, *Cultural Nationalism in Colonial Korea, 1920–1925* (Seattle: University of Washington Press, 1988).

13. Kenneth Wells, "The Nation, the World, and the Dissolution of the Shin'ganhoe: Nationalist Historiography in South Korea," *Korean Studies* 25 (2001): 179–206.

14. See Mark Caprio, *Japanese Assimilation Policies in Colonial Korea, 1910–1945* (Seattle: University of Washington Press, 2009), esp. chapter 5.

15. Hiroyuki Tanaka, "North Korea: Understanding Migration to and from a Closed Country," *Migration Policy Institute*, January 7, 2008. https://www.migrationpolicy.org/article/north-korea-understanding-migration-and-closed-country.

16. In some cases, ROK troops exacerbated the suffering of Vietnamese. See Hoang Do, "The Forgotten History of South Korean Massacres in Vietnam," *The Diplomat*, May 15, 2020. https://thediplomat.com/2020/05/the-forgotten-history-of-south-korean-massacres-in-vietnam/; Dien Luong, "It's Time for South Korea to Acknowledge Its Atrocities in Vietnam," *Foreign Policy*, December 30, 2022. https://foreignpolicy.com/2022/12/30/vietnam-war-south-korea-massacres-history-diplomacy/; and Anthony Kuhn, "A Vietnam War Massacre Case from 1968 Forces a New Reckoning in South Korea," *Morning Edition*, National Public Radio, April 12, 2023. https://www.npr.org/2023/04/12/1167951366/south-korea-vietnam-war-massacre-court-case.

17. Osita G. Afoaku, "U.S. Foreign Policy and Authoritarian Regimes: Change and Continuity in International Clientelism," *Journal of Third World Studies* 17 (2000): 13–40.

18. Allison O'Connor and Jeanne Batalova, "Korean Immigrants in the United States," *Migration Policy Institute*, April 10, 2019. https://www.migrationpolicy.org/article/korean-immigrants-united-states-2017.

19. In 1969, Korean immigrant nurses founded their own organization, the Korean American Nurses Association of Southern Cali (KANASC), to "inspire and empower Korean American nurses through philanthropy, education, and friendship" (https://www.kanasc.org/about-us). For more about Korean immigrant nurses, see Ji-Young An, Sunkyung Cha, and Haeran Jang, "Factors Affecting Job Satisfaction of Immigrant Korean Nurses," *Journal of Transcultural Nursing* 27 (2014): 126–135; Kumsook Seo and Miyoung Kim, "Clinical Work

Notes—Chapter VI

Experience of Korean Immigrant Nurses in the U.S. Hospitals," *Journal of Korean Academy of Nursing* 46 (2016): 238–248; Kumsook Seo and Miyoung Kim, "Professional Identity of Korean Nurse Practitioners in the United States," *Journal of the American Association of Nurse Practitioners* 29 (2017): 195–202; and Angela Jun, Sue-Kyung Sohn, and Jung-Ah Lee, "Lived Experience of Korean Immigrant Nurse Practitioners," *Journal of Comprehensive Nursing Research and Care* 6 (2021). https://gexinonline.com/archive/journal-of-comprehensive-nursing-research-and-care/JCNRC-175.

20. Paulina Cachero, "From AIDS to Covid-19, America's Medical System Has a Long History of Relying on Filipino Nurses to Fight on the Frontlines," *Time*, May 30, 2021. https://time.com/6051754/history-filipino-nurses-us/. On the history of Filipina nurses, see Catherine Ceniza Choy, *Empire of Care: Nursing and Migration in Filipino American History* (Durham, NC: Duke University Press, 2003). See also Danny Shin Kai Ung et al., "Global Migration and Factors Influencing Retention of Asian Internationally Educated Nurses: A Systematic Review," *Human Resources for Health* 22 (2024). https://www.ncbi.nlm.nih.gov/pmc/articles/PMC10905872/.

21. Sam Greenspan, "11 Gorgeously Ironic Misspellings in Protest Signs," March 11, 2018. https://11points.com/11-gorgeously-ironic-misspellings-protest-signs/; "Long-Time Mayor Signs Off," *WBEZ Chicago*, October 18, 2007. https://www.wbez.org/eight-forty-eight/2007/10/18/long-time-mayor-signs-off; Mariana van Zeller, "Bilingual Border Cities Challenge Movement to Make English the Official Language," *Huffington Post*, February 2, 2012. https://www.huffpost.com/entry/english-official-language-border-bilingual_n_1249307.

22. Arthur Chu, "Breaking Out the Broken English," *Code Switch*, National Public Radio, July 31, 2014. https://www.npr.org/sections/codeswitch/2014/07/31/336380977/breaking-out-the-broken-english; Luis Noe-Bustamante,

Lauren Mora, and Neil G. Ruiz, "Where Asian Immigrants Face Language Challenges: Navigating Daily Life and Communicating in English," *Pew Research Center*, December 19, 2022. https://www.pewresearch.org/2022/12/19/where-asian-immigrants-face-language-challenges-a-anavigating-daily-life-and-communicating-in-english/.

23. Jason Park, "Is English Taught in Korea?" *The Korean Guide*, August 18, 2022. https://thekoreanguide.com/is-english-taught-in-korea/; United States Forces Korea. https://www.usfk.mil/; and "U.S. Military Families in South Korea? Top U.S. General Wants Policy Change," *Korea Times*, December 4, 2020. https://www.koreatimes.co.kr/www/nation/2022/07/103_300367.html.

24. "If the prince have [sic] great faults, they ought to remonstrate with him, and if he do [sic] not listen to them after they have done so again and again, they ought to dethrone him." *The Works of Mencius*, in James Legge, trans., *The Four Books: Confucian Analects, The Great Learning, The Doctrine of the Mean, and the Works of Mencius* (China: The Commercial Press LTD, 19--?.), 847–848. Available at the Internet Archive, https://archive.org/details/fourbooksconfuci00leggiala/ and Chinese Text Project, https://ctext.org/mengzi/wan-zhang-ii.

25. *Analects of Confucius*, 2:15, in Legge, trans., *Four Books*, 19, and Chinese Text Project. https://ctext.org/analects.

Chapter VI

1. Biographical information about Florence Nightingale in this chapter was drawn largely from Edward Cook, *The Life of Florence Nightingale: Vol. 1 (1820–1861)* (London: Macmillan, 1913; Alpha Editions, 2020).

2. "Miss Nightingale Dies, Aged Ninety," *New York Times*, August 15, 1910, 7.

3. Florence Nightingale, Barbara Montgomery, Louise C. Selanders, Deva-Marie Beck, and Alex Attewell, *Florence Nightingale Today: Healing, Leadership,*

Global Action (Silver Spring: American Nurses Association, 2005), 288.
  4. *Ibid.*, 66.
  5. Jean C. Whelan, "American Nursing: An Introduction to the Past," in "Nursing, History, and Health Care," online in *PennNursing, University of Pennsylvania*, 2011. https://www.nursing.upenn.edu/nhhc/.
  6. Cook, *The Life of Florence Nightingale*, vol. 1, 468–490.
  7. *Ibid.*, 3–22.
  8. *Ibid.*, 104–115.
  9. *Ibid.*, 145–147.
  10. *Ibid.*, 148–150.
  11. *Ibid.*, 158–183.
  12. *Ibid.*, 177.
  13. *Ibid.*, 215–216, 266.
  14. *Ibid.*, 302–304.
  15. *Ibid.*, 314–315, 429–430.
  16. *Ibid.*, 439–455. Quotations on pp. 439–440.
  17. *Ibid.*, 362–366.

Afterword

  1. See Mireille Kingma, *Nurses on the Move: Migration and the Global Health Care Economy* (Ithaca: Cornell University Press, 2006).
  2. *Ibid.*, 2.
  3. Michelle Freeman et al., "Migration: A Concept Analysis from a Nursing Perspective," *Journal of Advanced Nursing* 68 (2012): 1176–1186.
  4. For example, Mireille Kingma, "Nurses on the Move: A Global Overview," *Health Services Research* 42 (2007): 1281–1298; Mireille Kingma, "Nurse Migration and the Global Health Care Economy," *Policy, Politics & Nursing Practice* 9 (2008): 328–333; Barbara L. Nichols et al., "An Integrative Review of Global Nursing Workforce Issues," *Annual Review of Nursing Research* 28 (2010): 113–132.
  5. "Asian American and Pacific Islander Heritage Month: May 2022," *United States Census Bureau*, April 18, 2022. https://www.census.gov/newsroom/facts-for-features/2022/asian-american-pacific-islander.html.
  6. Neil G. Ruiz and Abby Budiman, "Key Facts About Asian Americans, a Diverse and Growing population," *Pew Research Center*, April 29, 2021. https://www.pewresearch.org/fact-tank/2021/04/29/key-facts-about-asian-americans.
  7. "Nurses Flock to the United States in Search of Better Conditions and Pay," *JoongAng Daily*, December 25, 2023. https://koreajoongangdaily.joins.com/news/2023-12-25/national/socialAffairs/Nurses-flock-to-the-United-States-in-search-of-better-conditions-and-pay/1943674.
  8. Eunjoo Lee and Mikyung Moon, "Korean Nursing Students' Intention to Migrate Abroad," *Nurse Education Today* 33 (2013): 1517–1522.
  9. "Wŏllammin," *Hanguk minjok munhwa daebaekgwa* [Encyclopedia of Korean culture]. https://terms.naver.com/entry.naver?docId=572596&cid=46634&categoryId=46634.
  10. Kang Jeong-gu, "Haebang hu wŏllamin ŭi wŏllam tonggi wa kyegŭpsŏng e kwanhan yŏn'gu [A study on the motivation and class characteristics of Vietnamese people after liberation]," in *Han'guk chŏnjaeng kwa han'guk sahoe pyŏndong* [The Korean War and changes in Korean society], ed. Korean Sociological Association (Seoul: P'ulbit, 1992), 96–98; Kim Kwiok, *Wŏllamin ŭi saenghwal kyŏnghŏm kwa chŏngch'esŏng: Mit'ŭrobut'ŏ ŭi wŏllamin yŏn'gu* [Life experiences and identity of *wŏllamin*: A study of *wŏllamin* from below] (Seoul: Seoul National University Press, 1999); Kim Kwiok, "Wŏllamin ŭi saenghwal kyŏnghŏm kwa chŏngch'esŏng: mit'ŭrobut'ŏ ŭi wŏllamin yŏn'gu [Wŏllamin settled in Seoul after liberation]," *Chŏnnongsaron* 9 (2003): 61–90.
  11. John P. Dimoia, *Reconstructing Bodies: Biomedicine, Health, and Nation. Building in South Korea Since 1945* (Stanford: Stanford University Press, 2013).
  12. *Ibid.*, 16.
  13. Ji Yeon-ok, "Pet'ŭnam chŏnjaeng ch'amjŏn han'guk kun kanho changgyo ŭi kanho kyŏnghŏm [Nursing experience of Korean military nurses who

Notes—Afterword

participated in the Vietnam War]," *Kunjin kanho yŏn'gu* 23 (2005): 1–21.

14. Han Jung-jin, "Yŏsŏng kanho changgyo ŭi pet'ŭnam chŏnjaeng ch'amjŏn ch'ehŏm [A female nursing officer's experience participating in the Vietnam War]," PhD diss., Ewha Womans University, 2017; Jung-jin Han, "The Lived Experience of Korean Female Military Nursing Officers During the Vietnam War," *Journal of Transcultural Nursing* 30 (2019): 471–477.

15. Paul Ong, Lucie Cheng, and Leslie Evans, "Migration of Highly Educated Asians and Global Dynamics," *Asian and Pacific Migration Journal* 1 (1992): 543–545; Wilawan Kanjanapan, "The Immigration of Asian Professionals to the United States: 1988–1990," *International Migration Review* 29 (1995): 7–32; Lucie Cheng and Philip Q. Yang, "Global Interaction, Global Inequality, and Migration of the Highly Trained to the United States," *International Migration Review* 32 (1998): 626–653.

16. See Justus M. Van der Kroef, "The U.S. and the World's Brain Drain," *International Journal of Comparative Sociology* 11 (1970): 220–239; Judith A. Fortney, "International Migration of Professionals," *Population Studies* 24 (1970): 217–232; John M. Liu, "The Contours of Asian Professional, Technical and Kindred Work Immigration, 1965–1988," *Sociological Perspectives* 35 (1992): 673–704.

17. For example, between 1972 and 1985, the number of Filipino nurses (20,482) surpassed those of other Asian highly educated laborers in nine different occupations. On post–1965 Filipino immigration to the United States, see Charles B. Keely, "Philippine Migration: International Movement and Immigration to the United States," *International Migration Review* 7 (1973): 177–187; Monica Boyd, "The Changing Nature of Central and Southeast Asian Immigration to the United States: 1961–1972," *International Migration Review* 8 (1974): 507–519; Peter Smith, "The Social Demography of Filipino Migrations Abroad," *International Migration Review* 10 (1976): 307–353; James P. Allen, "Recent Immigration from the Philippines and Filipino Communities in the United States," *Geographical Review* 67 (1977): 195–208; Benjamin V. Cariño, "The Philippines and Southeast Asia: Historical Roots and Contemporary Linkages," in *Pacific Bridges: The New Immigration from Asia and The Pacific Islands*, ed. James T. Fawcett and Benjamin V. Cariño (Staten Island: Center for Migration Studies, 1987), 305–325.

18. Catherine Ceniza Choy, *Empire of Care: Nursing and Migration in Filipino American History* (Durham, NC: Duke University Press, 2003).

19. Yong-Suk Jung, "Beyond the Bifurcated Myth: The Medical Migration of Female Korean Nurses to West Germany in the 1970s," *Korean Journal of Medical History* 27 (2018): 225–266; In-Jin Yoon, *On My Own: Korean Businesses and Race Relations in America* (Chicago: University of Chicago Press, 1997).

20. As a result of the first agreement, 3,744 nurses and 3,289 nurse aides left for Germany from 1971 to 1974. See Lee Ae-joo et al., *P'adokkanho: p'yonggasaop ch'oejongbogoso* [The final report of the evaluation on the Germany-dispatched nurse projects] (Seoul: Malgeun, 2011), 89.

21. The president of the Deutsche Krankenhausgesellschaft raised objections to this report, concerned that hiring foreign nurses would tarnish the reputation of German hospitals. Yong-Suk Jung, "Beyond the Bifurcated Myth," 247–250.

22. In-Jin Yoon, *On My Own*, 6.

23. *Ibid.*, 165.

24. Song Ji-ho, "Segyehwa wa kanhosa ŭi haeoe ch'wiŏp [Globalization and overseas employment of nurses]," *Kanhohak t'amgu* 15 (2006): 18–34.; Cho Ho Soon Michelle, Cho Mi-gyeong, and Lee Gyeong-eun, "T'eksasŭ hanin kanho sahoe hyŏngsŏng kwa miju hanin sahoe e taehan konghŏn [The emergence of the North Texas Korean American Nurses Society and its contributions to Korean immigrant societies in the United States]," *Kanho haengjŏng hak'oeji* 17 (2011): 402–412; Eunjoo Lee

and Mikyung Moon, "Korean Nursing Students' Intention to Migrate Abroad," 1517–1522; Kumsook Seo and Miyoung Kim, "Clinical Work Experience of Korean Immigrant Nurses in U.S. Hospitals," *Journal of Korean Academy of Nursing* 46 (2016): 238–248; Helen Kim, "'My Life Would Have Been Happier in Germany': Korean Guestworker Nurses' Journeys to Germany and to the U.S.," *Identities: Global Studies in Culture and Power* 30 (2023): 823–840.

25. For example, see Hong Sin-yeong, *Han'guk kanho yŏksa* [Korean nursing history] (Seoul: Hyŏnmunsa, 2004); Ok Seong-deuk, *Han'guk kŭndae kanho yŏksa hwabojip* [Korean modern nursing history photobook] (Seoul: Taehan kanho hyŏp'oe, 2012); Sin Mi-ja et al., *Kanho ŭi yŏksa* [Nursing history] (Seoul: Korean Nurses Association Press, 2013); Yonsei University College of Nursing History Committee, *Yŏnse kanho: Han'guk kanho kyoyuk ŭi san yŏksa* [Yonsei nursing: A living history of nursing education in Korea] (Seoul: Yonsei University College of Nursing History Committee, 2019).

26. For information of Korean participation in the Vietnam War, see Academy of Korean Studies, ed., *1960nyŏndae ŭi taeoe kwan'gye wa nambuk munje* [Foreign relations and inter-Korean issues in the 1960s] (Sungnam: Baeksan Seodang, 1999); Yun Chung-ro, *Pet'ŭnam kwa han'guk ŭi pan'gong tokchae kukka hyŏngsŏngsa* [History of the formation of anti-communist dictatorships in Vietnam and Korea] (Seoul: Sŏnin, 2005); Yun Chung-ro, "P'awŏl kisulcha ŭi pet'ŭnam chŏnjaeng kyŏnghŏm kwa saenghwal segye pyŏnhwa [Vietnam War experience and life world changes of engineers dispatched to Vietnam]," *Sahoe wa yŏksa* 71 (2006): 217–250; Yun Chung-ro, "Pet'ŭnam chŏnjaeng shigi han mi wŏl kwan'gye esŏ han'guk ŭi chŏngch'esŏng mandŭlgi [Creating Korean identity in Korea–U.S.–Vietnam Relations During the Vietnam War]," *Tamnon* 201 (2007): 171–203; Kim Gyeong-hui, "Troops Sent to Vietnam and Economic Effects [*Wŏllam p'abyŏng kwa kyŏngje hyogwa*]," MA thesis, Kyungpook National University, 2008; Yun Chung-ro, *Pet'ŭnam chŏnjaeng ŭi han'guk sahoesa: It'in chŏnjaeng, oraedoen hyŏnjae* [Korean social history of the Vietnam War: Forgotten war, old present] (Seoul: P'urŭn yŏksa, 2015); Park Tae-gyun, *Pet'ŭnam chŏnjaeng: It'yŏjin chŏnjaeng, pantchok ŭi kiŏk* [Vietnam War: A forgotten war, half a memory] (Seoul: Han'gyŏre ch'ulp'an, 2015); Lee Sin-jae, "Pet'ŭnam chŏnjaenggi han'gukkun t'aegwŏndo kyogwandan ŭi p'abyŏng kwa yŏk'al [Dispatch and role of Korean military taekwondo instructors during the Vietnam War]," *Kukkiwŏn t'aegwŏndo yŏn'gu* 8 (2017): 51–52; Cho Seo-yeon, "1960 nyŏndae pet'ŭnam chŏnjaeng yŏnghwa wa p'awŏl han'gukkun ŭi namsŏngsŏng [The masculinity of the Korean army in 1960s Vietnam War films]," *Minjok munhaksa yŏn'gu* 68 (2018): 495–496; Cho Seo-yeon, "Han'guk 'pet'ŭnam chŏnjaeng 'ŭi chŏngch'i wa yŏnghwajŏk chaehyŏn [Politics and cinematic representation of the Korean 'Vietnam War']," *Han'guk kŭngnyesul yŏn'gu* 69 (2020): 241–244; Ministry of Defense Military Compilation Research Institute, (*Chŭngŏn ŭl t'onghae pon*) *pet'ŭnam chŏnjaeng kwa han'gukkun* [(Viewed through testimony) Vietnam War and Korean army] (Seoul: Ministry of Defense Military Compilation Research Institute, 2023); Byung-Kook Kim and Ezra F. Vogel, eds., *The Park Chung Hee Era: The Transformation of South Korea* (Cambridge, MA: Harvard University Press, 2011).

27. Ministry of Health and Social Affairs, "P'awŏl ŭiryodan ch'ŏl [The collection of the medical team deployed to Vietnam]," National Archives of Korea, South Korea.

28. Academy of Korean Studies, *Wŏllammin kusul saengaesa chosa yŏn'gu* [Survey of oral life history of *wollammin*]. http://waks.aks.ac.kr/rsh/?rshID=AKS-2014-KFR-1230004.

Index

Numbers in ***bold italics*** refer to pages with illustrations

American Association of Colleges of Nursing 10
American Nurses Association 4, 9

Bible 51, 65, 73, 106–107, 115, 119
Bucheon 67
Buddhism 42, 95
Busan 30, 50

capitalism 13, 15
China ***30***, 31, 37, 45, 50
Choy, Catherine Ceniza (author of *Empire of Care: Nursing and Migration in Filipino American History*) 155–156
Christianity 26, 32, 41, 42, 46, 65, 72, 105–107, 127, 153, 161
class 7, 17, 44–45, 48, 53, 56, 102, 115, 157, 159
Cold War 16, 22
collaboration 15–16
comfort women 16
Communism 13–14, 20–21, 34–35, 41, 46, 85, 94–95, 151
Confucianism 17, 25, 44, 58, 63, 70, 129–130, 137, 151
Cook, Edward (author of *The Life of Florence Nightingale Vol. 1 (1820–1861)*) 121
Covid 1, 23, 146
Crimean War 118, 120–122

Daegwon (Daegwon-dong) ***30***, 31–37, 41, 43, 47
democracy 21, 34, 85, 94
DiMoia, John (author of *Reconstructing Bodies: Biomedicine, Health, and Nation-Building in South Korea Since 1945*) 154

Eastern University 125, 127–129, 139–140
Ewha Womans University 21, 58, 59, 61–64, 141–142

faith 36, 46–47, 65, 79, 105–106, 119, 140, 161
Federal Nurse Training Act of 1964 9
Ford, Betty 108–***109***

Gaeseong 42, 50
gender roles 6, 17, 45, 118, 123, 129, 151, 155
George, Julie B. (author of *Nursing Theories: The Base for Professional Nursing Practice*) 123
globalization 141, 149

Han 21

Immigration and Nationality Act of 1965 155
imperialism 15, 19–21, 160
International Council of Nursing 141

Jangdan 40, 42, 50
January 4 Retreat 50
Japan 3, 14, 17–21; occupation by/imperial rule 14–15, 18–19, 31–32, 34–35, 42, 94, 98
Jeong-jin, Han 155
Ji, Yeon-ok 154–155
Jinhae 54
Jung, Yong-Suk (author of "Beyond the

171

Index

Bifurcated Myth: The Medical Migration of Female Korean Nurses to West Germany in the 1970s") 156–158

Kang, Jung-Koo 153
Kim Il-sung 13–15, 36, 61, 70
Kim Jong-il 13
Kim, Kwi-ok 153
Kim, Seongbo 159–160
Kim, Tae Won (mother of Sung Yoo) 31–33, 36–39, 45, 51, 53, 61, 68, 70–72
Kim Jong-un 13
Korea Overseas Development Corporation 8
Korean Communist Party 14
Korean language 34, 62–63
Korean War 16, 46–50

language barrier 8–9, 17, 23–24, 83, 86, 91–92, 96–97, 100–104, 107, 110–111, 128, 131, 133
Lee, Yuen Kuen (father of Sung Yoo) 31–32, 44, 47, 50–53, 119–120
liberal arts education 10, 112, 118, 127, 144

MacArthur, Douglas 49
Medicaid 9, 107–108, 110
Medicare 9, 108, 110
Mogpo 32, 46, 48, 50, 52

National Council Licensure Examination (NCLEX) 129, 131, 150
National Institute for Nursing Research 9
National Institutes of Health 9, 71
neocolonialism 22
Nightingale, Florence 5, 7, 11, 25, 29, 74, 115, 116–126, 138–140; publications 118–119, 125
North Korea (Democratic People's Republic of Korea) 13, *30*, 34–39, 42, 46, 151; military 46–48; prejudice against 44, 48, 70, 85, 152
nurse migration 149–151, 154–161
nursing: development as a profession 5–7, 116–117, 122–123, 138; education 5–9, 25, 59, 62, 82, 96, 99, 104, 127–128; ethics 9–10, 26; stigma against 7–8, 26, 29, 56–58, 93, 117, 132, 136, 150; theory 25, 114–115, 117–118, 123, 127, 139, 146–147

106th General Hospital, Yokohama 3, 11

Partition of Korea 17, 21, 34, 36
Patient Rights Law 124
P'awŏl ŭiryodan ch'ŏ ("The collection of the medical team deployed to Vietnam") 159
People's committees 15
Philippines 155–156
poverty 6, 14, 43, 48, 53, 59, 64–65, 72, 107–108
Princeton, New Jersey 111, 142
Princeton Medical Center 113, 115, 123–125
Protectorate regime 19
Pyongyang *30*, 37

refugee 13–14, 32, 35–38, 40, 42–44, 46, 50, 52
reunification of Korea 13, 16
Russia 13–14, 19–20, 38

Saigon (Ho Chi Minh) *75*–76, *78*–79, 87, 94
Seoul 18, *30*, 42, 46, 48–50, 54, 67–68, 71, 141–142
South Korea (Republic of Korea) 15, 17, 23, *30*, 34, 46, 67, 108; military 40, 47, 50, 87–*88*, 154–155; prejudice against 15–17, 45
Soviet Union 16, 21
Suncheon 50–52
Sung Duk (younger brother of Sung Yoo) 33, 36, 38, 45, 54, 68
Sung Hee (oldest brother of Sung Yoo) 33, 46, 50
Sung Kul (older brother of Sung Yoo) 33, 42, 45, 47, 49, 52, 54, 56–57, 61, 63, 65, 68–71, 96, 116–117, 140, 146
Sung Sook (older sister of Sung Yoo) 33, 50, 52

Tet Offensive 3
38th parallel 21, *30*, 36–38, 50, 151
Treaty on Comprehensive Strategic Partnership 13
Tuy Hoa *75*, 79–80, 87, 90

United States 16, 22, 49, 57–58, 107, 111, 150, 154–157; culture 10, 27, 86, 95, 101–102, 109–110, 112–113, 130, 134, 144–145; military 40, 49, 89–91, 108
U.S. Army Nurse Corps 3

Index

Vietcong 22, 73, 81, 83–84
Vietnam 3, 21–22, 74–*78*, 85, 94; partition of 75, 94–95
Vietnam War 3, 21–22, 71–73, 77–79, 85, 95, 154–155
Villanova University 114, 139
Visiting Nurse Association 104, 108

Wald, Lillian 7
Washington, D.C. 10, 99, 104, 106–107
White Horse Division 87–88
White House 108, *109*, 110
Wŏllammin 151–153, 158–160
Workers' Party of Korea 14
World Health Organization 67, 71
World War II 5, 8, 20–21, 31, 34, 36, 49, 98

Yoo, Hans (son of Sung Yoo) 113
Yoo, Hyen Ju "Julie" (older daughter of Sung Yoo) 71, *93*, 101
Yoo, Hyo Min "Peggy" (younger daughter of Sung Yoo) *93*, 97–98, 104–106
Yoo, Insok "Len" (husband of Sung Yoo) 64–66, 68–69, *93*, 96–97, 100–101, *146*
Yoon, In-Jin (author of *On My Own: Korean Businesses and Race Relations in America*) 156–158
Young Kyu (mother-in-law of Sung Yoo) 64, 69–70, 71, 74, 92, 97, 104–106, 111

www.ingramcontent.com/pod-product-compliance
Ingram Content Group UK Ltd.
Pitfield, Milton Keynes, MK11 3LW, UK
UKHW042015140426
5217IPUK00015B/1185